#SleeveLife

LOSING HALF OF MYSELF
AND FINDING THE REST

Jonathan Dichter

SleeveLife, LLC
Bothell, WA

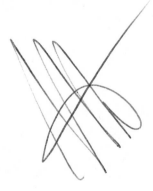

Jonathan Dichter I SleeveLife, LLC
PO Box 14564
Mill Creek, WA 98082
www.SleeveLifeBook.com

Book Layout ©2017 BookDesignTemplates.com
Cover Design ©2018 BucklinHillCovers.com
Edited by: Jennifer DeLucy - jenniferdelucy@gmail.com

Ordering Information:
Quantity sales. Special discounts are available on quantity
purchases by corporations, associations, and others. For details, contact the address above.

#SleeveLife/Jonathan Dichter. — Print — 1st ed.
ISBN 978-1-7321321-0-8

Contents

FIRST FOREWORD
By Dr. Catherine Zeh

It may be the deepest dream of most physicians that their patients actually follow their medical advice, but this is certainly true of primary care physicians such as myself. Despite many years of training in the art and science of medicine, I often feel that my most critical role is that of educator. The men, women, and children who come to me as patients lead complex lives and come from a wide variety of social, educational, and economic backgrounds. If my patients don't understand how their bodies work, they are less able to grasp details of disease process and treatment, much less follow through on a path towards healing. It is up to me to discern how best to engage my patients in order to guide them to healthier lives.

Sometimes this process of engagement spans many years. When I first met Jonathan, he was focused less on his own health and more on the needs of his aging parents and growing family. This is often a balancing act, deferring one's own needs for a time, but a reckoning must eventually come. In fits and starts, Jonathan gradually faced the threats to his own health and happiness, and we spent long visits talking about treatment options. Over this time, we developed a shared respect and trust that seemed to provide the foundation for him to take the great leap towards bariatric surgery.

It has been a great joy, as a physician, to follow Jonathan's experience and successes. I know that this great investment of time, energy, and resources on his part will help ensure a longer, healthier, happier life for him. I find I am especially appreciative, though, of Jonathan's willingness to share his experience with others. While I hope to educate my patients, I know that some days I learn even more from them and their experiences. I am a better physician for having worked with Jonathan on this quest. I congratulate him!

SECOND FOREWORD
By Dr. Robert Landerholm

Jonathan Dichter is courageous.

Some might think he proved this by completing law school and starting his private practice. But that is not so much an act of courage as it is personal and academic achievement. Perhaps his being an actor and comic, going on stage live in front of people, would impress some as courageous. As an ancient comic purportedly said, "Dying is easy, comedy is hard." Or perhaps Jonathan in writing this book portrayed courage. Paraphrasing Churchill it takes a certain fortitude, audacity, boldness to "fling" one's completed work to the mercy and scrutiny of the public. But none of these are illustrative of the courage Jonathan has shown to me.

Jonathan has a disease. That disease is called obesity. To see him now, you wouldn't know it. But he knows it, those closest to him know it. I know it. And it was killing him. Yet he had the courage to face it and do something about it.

Like Jonathan, people who suffer with this disease have years, even decades taken from them. And certainly they're made miserable in the process. Most try very hard to do something about it. They diet, exercise, count calories, get personal trainers, spend in some cases thousands of dollars "to get better." Most succeed for a time, losing weight, feeling better. But then, in the vast majority of cases, the weight comes back plus extra. That's the true, killer nature of this disease. Hand in glove come the unfortunate medical problems ... high blood pressure, elevated cholesterol, diabetes, sleep apnea, joint aches, and so on that take their toll. And, to quite literally add insult to injury, the disease is a very public one, unhidden from friends, family, coworkers, even strangers we pass on the street.

Jonathan was slowly and definitely dying. Many who suffer like Jonathan, for whatever reason, seem content to die younger than they should. But he chose to face his killer, learn, and do something extraordinary. Something many would consider "extreme and risky." That took courage. The courage of a life time.

I've had the good pleasure of getting to know Jonathan, professionally and personally. By seeing his success and the success of people like him, my own life is enriched. I often tell my patients "I get to live vicariously" by what they positively experience in their lives. This has never been more true than with Jonathan. The stories I get to hear almost daily of achievement and happiness, from the audacious to the sublime, make my professional life full. How could you not revel in people getting healthier, stronger, living the life they want to live? By no means is the process a panacea or necessarily easy. It takes work, dedication, focus, and energy to make it happen. And, like Jonathan, it takes courage.

I read Jonathan's book #Sleevelife a little over a year after my own weight loss surgery. I couldn't help but wish that it had been in my hands before my own decision to have the gastric sleeve. Jonathan's honesty about the struggles coming to his decision to have surgery were similar to my own and would've offered the assurance I needed. This book is a great reminder that we aren't alone and offers the motivation needed to take the next step.
—JENNIFER, WEIGHT LOSS SURGERY PATIENT

#Sleevelife is like sitting down with a warm cup of protein coffee and a close friend. Jonathan shares his story in a completely real, transparent, and vulnerable way that I completely resonate with as a fellow sleever six years post-surgery. All of the emotions, the anxiety, the changes, the adjustments....he leaves nothing out. Jonathan's book would prepare someone considering weight loss surgery better than any surgeon or counselor ever could. I'd prescribe reading it before having surgery, and then re-reading it probably once a month (or as needed) after surgery! You can't help but relate and feel like you've got a friend along for the journey, inspiring you every step of the way.
—ROBIN, WEIGHT LOSS SURGERY PATIENT

Jonathan does a wonderful job sharing his journey leading up to weight loss surgery and subsequently the successes and challenges that came after. His

This book is lovingly dedicated to:

Kathryn Dichter
Elizabeth Dichter
Dr. Catherine Zeh
Dr. Robert Landerholm
Dayna Pitsch
Jennifer DeLucy

I could not have done this without you.

Introduction

So, here's the thing, I'm a fat guy. I've been (I was?) a fat guy for a really long time. And I'm finally tired enough with that to just do something about it. Oh, I've done things about it before. I've tried Weight Watchers, the Atkins diet, Body-for-Life, brown rice, grapefruit, weight training, eating nothing but bamboo, and everything else you've ever heard of trying. Now it's time to try something else. Something drastic: weight loss surgery. I admit it—I am terrified. But I figured you might be terrified too, and maybe in the same situation. And there's no sense in us going through this without each other. Okay, well, there's no sense in you going through this without me since I've already gone through it and have had the success you can see on the cover of the book. (The funny thing is I'm writing this introduction just a few days after making the decision to have surgery in the first place, but I'm assuming that if I don't have success enough to put a picture on the front of the book nobody's going to read it. So talk about betting on success!) I figured we could do this together. Because whether it's surgery, a weight-loss journey, or some other major life transition you're about to go through, nothing will help it more than going through it with someone who has been through it and who is really damn funny. So strap in my friend, and I will walk you through the highs and lows of my weight-loss surgery story, starting with the lows: my weight loss history, and a tale of how I got to where I am today—A 38 year old successful attorney single dad...who weighs (weighed?) four hundred and five pounds.

CHAPTER 1

Credentials and Qualifications

Before we get into the nitty gritty of how this all goes and what happens as you decide to have surgery, we should have a little bit of a frank talk. I mean, who the heck am I to tell you about my weight-loss journey? Well, dear reader, I'm glad you asked. I present to you here my "dieting" resume, as it were.

I wasn't always fat. In fact, I was a skinny, active kid. I climbed every rock I could find and biked everywhere, I played little league. But as I got into middle school I started growing...in all sizes. So much so that at my junior high they demanded I play football because I was two inches taller and fifty pounds heavier than anyone else. They wrote "TANK" across my helmet and put me on the defensive line. This was humorous in itself as I'd grown up in a family that didn't watch football. We watched baseball.

> *"Okay coach, what do I do?"*
> *"Look for the ball. Then go get it."*
> *"What if someone has it?"*
> *"Knock him down."*

This seemed like a reasonable plan of action until about four games into the season when I took a helmet to the left knee and snapped my growth plate in half. Thus ended my football career and began my speech and debate career. The more sedentary extra curricular. Great. I already shared the struggles my parents had with weight, and now a more sedentary lifestyle wasn't going to do me any favors.

We tried diets at home together from time to time. The earliest "diet" memory I have is from high school. I couldn't tell you my weight but I think I was around a size 42 waist. In fact I'm sure of it because some upperclassmen (I was in accelerated anatomy and physiology with seniors) bet me I couldn't get down to a 36 waist. What I didn't know was how much they were actually making fun of me behind my back. Which brings me to teasing. Let's get this out of the way first. If you tease fat people, you're a grade-A, certified asshat. Being overweight isn't about lack of control, nor stupidity, nor laziness. Do you think a third of America doesn't know how to "diet and exercise" and is just stupid? No. Most of us know how. But we can't make it work. We try and sometimes we succeed. But other times we fail. And that makes it worse. Because then not only do we feel physically lousy, we know we failed too. So now we're not just fat, we're a fat failure. For many of us, it's the thing about which we are most sensitive and hardest on ourselves. And when you aim squarely at that soft target, my friend, you're simply stabbing us through our hearts as surely as if you used an actual knife. Many of us fight back with humor. Some with fists. Some just repress it and get depressed. Incidentally some of us through our lives (myself included) have done all three.

Depression when you're overweight sucks. Depression about being overweight is damn near impossible to get a handle on by yourself. Imagine how this works. You start thinking awful things about yourself, none of which are even remotely true, of course.

I feel lousy about myself. Nobody will ever love me. I'm fat and ugly. I can't seem to control it. I CAN control how much food I put in my mouth, and Ben and Jerry love me. So I'll have this ice cream. And now that the pint is gone I realize that I've just done something to make myself even heavier, which makes me feel worse about myself. And so on and so forth. (Hey—I know I promised laughs, but some of this shit just ain't funny).

Anyway, let's get back to the diets we tried as a family in high school. The first one I remember was Richard Simmons' all new "Deal-a-Meal". I thought this would be fun because it involved brightly colored cards and looked a bit like a really strange game of Magic: the Gathering. Sadly, the cumbersome cards and exchanges and portions left poor Richard's plan not all that user friendly to my family, and we abandoned it quickly. *Hey! We're free! Ice cream time!*

Around about the time I got my driver's license I was up to 280 pounds. At six-foot-two and broad framed, I carried it well, but I knew I was wearing 2XLs for the most part. I think this was when my father, an overweight doctor, brought home the first copy I'd ever seen of Dr. Atkins' book, the New Diet Revolution.

At the time he decided we would try it together, but not my mother. I got the impression that somehow he was worried about the way all the protein would affect a woman's body and we were kind of like guinea pigs. That first version of Atkins preached no carbs and all the fat and meat you wanted. We made fried chicken, ate entire blocks of cheese, had 10 egg omelettes with bacon, avoided those poisonous carbs (like apples, oranges and grapes), and lost about 5 pounds over like 3 months. Clearly there needed to be balance in this diet too. Balance and, apparently, discipline.

I met a guy in my law school section named Joey. Joey was *strong*. And I mean *STRONG*. And he liked working out. I'd also stumbled upon a book called *Body-for-LIFE*. This book encouraged you to enter a body transformation challenge for twelve weeks, showing you all sorts of ripped and buff people on the covers and their twelve week transformations. Yours could end up in the book too, and even end up with you being a paid spokesman for a sports supplement company! Okay - I doubted I'd win the prize, but the program seemed solid. Between working out with Joey and eating right and lifting a lot of weights, I lost about 68 pounds in twelve weeks. I felt great. But try as I might I was never able to duplicate the successes I had those first twelve weeks. Then I finished law school and started dating the woman who'd become my ex wife eventually and the weight came right back. Plus some more.

CHAPTER 2

RunDisney – An Obsession Begins

In 2007 I heard about a friend who was getting in shape to run the Walt Disney World Half Marathon. You actually get to run *through* the castle. At the time (and my whole life before and since) I was kind of a Disney nerd so this sounded amazing. But there's no way I could do it. I needed help and support. Fortunately I was the cohost of a somewhat popular Disney themed Podcast. And so I announced that I'd be running and raising money for charity - specifically the Make a Wish foundation, my go to charity of choice. (If you're curious why, yes, diseases are awful, but cures can be years and decades away, and I want to do something to make a sick kid happy and brighten their life *today.* End of public service announcement.)

You know, sitting here recalling that moment when I heard my friend detail that he would be running and the days and weeks leading to my decision, I'm struck by the fact that if I'd never heard him that day, I might not be here writing this for you. So much of this story is woven into RunDisney (highs and lows) and I really didn't realize it until I thought about it. So thanks, Lou! More on those highs and lows in a minute or ten.

The additional support of Weight Watchers online helped me lose over 85 pounds in about six months. I went from barely being able to walk a mile to walking over ten miles. In January 2009, I completed my first half-marathon at Walt Disney World. At mile ten, I realized every step I took was one further than I'd ever taken before.

I saw a man wearing a great t-shirt. "I'm old, I'm slow, so what?" This made me smile, and I scooted over to say hi. It turned out the shirt was produced by my favorite running columnist. The man wearing it? The very same person. I was floored. I asked if I could tell him my story, which I did. He asked me to make him two promises: 1) Never stop telling my story and 2) Now that I knew how healthy felt, never go back. I promised both (and ironically, although I struggled with promise number two, I'm still keeping it better than ever before). When I crossed that first finish line I literally exploded with emotion. I don't think I stopped crying for nearly 20-30 minutes.

Eight months later, in September 2009, I ran the Disneyland Half Marathon. This was a truly momentous run, as I'd recently started my own business, and moved my parents cross country while finding out I was going to be a father, and through all of that, still managed to go down and do it. I was nowhere near as fast, because I was heavier already, but I finished.

The next year brought me a finisher's medal for the Walt Disney World Princess Half Marathon, but my pacing was getting slower and slower as my waist was getting bigger and bigger again.

That fall, I attempted the inaugural Walt Disney World Wine and Dine Half Marathon. At mile seven my legs started to ache. At mile 8 they started to buckle. At mile nine I sat down for a moment. When a medic on a bike came by and asked if I was alright, I asked to be carted to the finish line. I wasn't sure how this had happened, but I was sure it wouldn't happen again. I was fooling myself and not willing to look at what changes I'd been making...and not making...until the 2011 Walt Disney World Half Marathon. During a RunDisney event, you are required to keep a certain pace - specifically a sixteen minute mile. If you can't keep that pace and are passed by the "pacers", you can be picked up by a bus and "swept" to the finish where, although you still get your medal, you did not complete the race.

The pacers are affectionately called the "balloon ladies". This is because there are three of them, they are female, and they wear large balloons tied to their waists. As you see them pass you it's the signal that you'd better hurry your butt up. On each race course, they are the last people to begin, so if you start a few thousand people ahead of them you have a buffer. There are, on average, three or four "sweep points," where, if you've fallen behind the balloon ladies", a bus will get you.

In 2011 as I felt my pace dwindle (I'd started at the front of my corral and thought I had a nice buffer available to me) and my side was hurting as badly as (if not more than) my feet, I saw them get past me. I tried to keep with them, but I couldn't. I could still *see* them, but they were ahead of me and I had literally no chance to catch them. This was about eight miles into a 13.1 mile walk, and nearly to the overpass used as a cloverleaf turn to get from World Drive to EPCOT, I actually watched the bus pull across the street in front of me. I knew that my race was over. And deep down something in me knew that my racing was over too. I sat on that bus feeling despondent. Then I had the audacity to wear the medal I paid for, but somehow didn't earn. Some people told me to wear it proudly. I'd paid for it and gone eight miles. But it said 13.1 on it. And some of my "runner" friends looked down on me for wearing it. Criticized me. A few even stopped talking to me for awhile.

I didn't even tell most of them I came down a year later for one more runDisney event in October 2011. I was determined to give it another try. I wasn't willing to give up. I also wasn't willing to train or prepare. I just wanted to go and do it again by sheer force of will. It was one of the hottest race days I'd ever been a part of, and I wasn't really prepared for it—the heat, or the race.

I worked my way into the front of my corral and knew that what I needed to do was run at the start as far as I could, so as to get as much space between me and those damn balloon ladies (who I'm sure are lovely people, despite their demonization by runDisney folk). And run I did. Fast and hard. Exhaustively for about three-quarters of a mile. Then, out of breath and pouring sweat, I slowed to my normal pace. By the time I reached mile nine, I knew for sure I would be able to finish this race. I also knew for sure that something was really really wrong. I figured I was tired and my body was just running on empty, literally. I was starting to see a little fuzzy and wheeze a little. My thoughts didn't even register that despite the heat and activity, I stopped sweating around mile seven.

I sojourned on, one foot in front of the other, until I finished. I have no pictures of me after that race, as I got my medal and bypassed photos entirely. In fact, I have no memory of walking to the monorail to get back to my resort. You see, what I hadn't accounted for was my excess weight (now around 70 pounds heavier than in 2009) and its need for excess water, not to mention the extreme heat. I was severely dehydrated, and had no idea. I just knew if I didn't sit down, I was likely to fall down. I staggered into an empty monorail car, and looked at the bench. When I sat, I felt immediately like I was going to be sick, and so the natural thing to do was put my head down and my feet up.

At that point, the world started spinning, and I think I blacked out momentarily. The monorail ride from EPCOT (where the race ended) back to the Transportation and Ticket Center takes about six minutes or so (about thirteen minutes round trip). I remember feeling us slowing down at the TTC and wanting to sit up and move. I had to get off this monorail to get on another one to go to my hotel. In fact, my plane home was leaving in six hours. I needed to get going. But alas, I couldn't budge my body. A quick glance around told me I was alone in this monorail car somehow (it was at the far end of the train). I tried speaking up, but only a small squeak came out. I was dry as a bone, and literally paralyzed. Also, I was scared out of my mind.

As the monorail pulled away from the TTC to go back to EP-COT, I remember wondering to myself whether or not I was actually going to die on this monorail and never see my daughter again. I wasn't being dramatic. I was terrified. I couldn't move and couldn't think straight. After two laps on the monorail laying there alone and scared, and frankly in and out of consciousness while the dehydration got worse and worse, we pulled into the TTC again, and a cast member happened to peek his head into the car and see me.

"Are you okay, sir?"

I managed to squeak out a "no".

"Water?"

"Yes."

In moments I was being helped to a seated position and being given water to sip. The first sips were like lifeblood flowing back into my body, and before I knew it I was being helped to my feet and sat in a wheelchair. I was wheeled by a cast member from one monorail platform to another. Yes, a half marathon finisher, complete with medal, wheezing and panting and being carted around on a wheelchair from place to place.

I finally managed to get enough energy and control to walk and found my way to a couch in a quiet corner of the hotel where I was staying, and collapsed until it was time to leave for my plane ride home. I cried openly there as I was between floors and nobody really was there to watch me. I was embarrassed—more so than when I'd been swept for some reason. I was also scared. My body hadn't cooperated and I'd nearly hurt myself as a result. Severely.

I believed at that point I was done with runDisney. I was giving up. I couldn't justify the expenses anymore when my body and mind clearly weren't up for the challenge. I'd reconsider—and fail once more—three years later.

CHAPTER 3

A Parade of Horribles

In 2009, an avalanche of bad tidings began to unfold. (Insert sufficiently creepy Michael Giacchino music here to give a sense of foreboding.) There is apparently the concept of the "major life event"—that thing which creates a dividing line in your world. There's you before "it" and you after "it". You'll usually go through nine to ten of these in a lifetime (think marriage, divorce, kids, deaths, job, etc). I went through nine in about eighteen months. I should mention that not all of the "major life events" I'm about to detail for you were negative experiences. But all of them were stressors. Massive ones.

Wait! Don't stop reading! This isn't some tale of woe or a call for sympathy about my problems. I promise. But many of us go through the same things and they can contribute to losing our grip and ability to control certain aspects of our lives. They cause stress. Stress causes problems with follow through. And as a result, the weight comes back. Which it did. And then some.

At this point I had been married for three years and my wife and I decided it was time to try for a family. Within a month, she was already pregnant. In April, as we were preparing to share the good news with our families, I got a call that would change nearly everything for the next year.

My father, who was my hero, had been struggling with failing health since the year 2000, when he'd had an emergency triple bypass and followed it with a post-operative stroke a week later. Since then he'd bounced back and forth out in and out of the hospital with pneumonias and other ailments. He'd developed congestive heart failure, had portions of his bowel seize up and be removed, and more over the years. My folks were living in rural Oklahoma at the time (and just for a moment, let's imagine a Brooklyn Jew and an Italian girl from Queens living in Rural Oklahoma), and here was my mother, on the phone with me shortly after my 31st birthday.

She was worried because my father, who for years had been the person to take care of everything for them (and I do mean everything. (She had to have a ninety-something-year-old neighbor show her how to put gas in the car when Dad was sick and had started to get confused.)

He'd been diagnosed with what's called vascular dementia. As his congestive heart failure worsened, the oxygen levels to his brain would decrease, and he'd get confused. It was bad when Mom and I had to have a talk with him about the fact that he wasn't allowed to be a doctor anymore.

Through my wife's pregnancy, I helped my father manage the sale of his medical practice and the sale of their home. In July 2009, I flew to Oklahoma to finalize the sales and put my mom, dad, and maternal grandmother (who was living with them) on an airplane to the Pacific Northwest where I'd selected a lovely assisted living retirement community for them —and within walking distance of my home. I figured I walked a lot now, since I'd just recently completed a runDisney event.

I also figured it was stressful being in Oklahoma and going through all that, so when the food of the day involved country fried everything, ice cream shakes, and desserts of every kind you can imagine, I thought that I'd be fine indulging. I also had other things on my mind.

You see, as the plane has landed in Oklahoma, I tried checking my work email. It seemed to be down. Four hours later I received an email to my personal account saying my law firm was laying me off because the boss had decided she could hire someone cheaper than me. This with zero notice and zero warning after having been the head of the criminal division at that firm for five years. I was officially unemployed and with a baby on the way. Did I mention we'd just furnished the nursery? Because we had. Our savings were gone.

Of course, in the midst of moving my family cross country, I immediately called every lawyer I knew asking for a job. Nobody had one to give; it was the summer of 2009. Remember that one? So when I got home and got Mom and Dad settled, I went to every bank in town. I figured I'd been a lawyer six years and was going to open a firm doing what I'd been building a reputation toward—getting a small business loan should be no problem.

"Your business plan is solid and your earning potential is high. As soon as you've been in business two years, we'll happily loan you anything you'd like." *Are you kidding me?!?*

Swallowing my pride, I requested, and was granted a small business loan from the first national bank of my grandma. If I hadn't been, I honestly don't know how I'd have survived the next few years. As it was, they were going to be hard enough on me.

Opening a business is a stressful occasion. Doing so with a newborn is damn near impossible. Doing so with a newborn while helping your aging parents (both of whom struggled with health issues and occasional stays in the hospital) settle into a new life at a retirement community was almost more than I could bear. Fast food was happening a lot. As was snacking. Lots of snacking. It was my stress coping mechanism of choice. Food never let me down.

On Valentine's Day 2010, my wife and I were away from our four-month-old daughter for the first time on a date. We were enjoying a night out when my phone rang. It was my mother. My father was headed back into the hospital after a fall, was confused, and was coughing like he had pneumonia.

One week later, he called a family meeting in the hospital.

"We all know I'm not getting any better. What's going to happen is this: I'm going to bounce in and out of the hospital every four to six months for the next two years or so and then my heart will give out and I'm going to die. That's not what I want. At all. I want my fluid restrictions lifted, my medication stopped, and I want to be kept comfortable."

We had our primary care doctor, Dr. Catherine Zeh (who you'll notice was one of the dedications in this book) evaluate him to make sure he was lucid. He was. He was lucid. Tired. Exhausted, in fact. But lucid.

It was at that moment that Dr. Zeh and I had the first conversation I've ever had with her that I know I'll remember forever. She told me by phone, calmly and with caring and what sounded like love in her heart (and you'll never tell me anything different about this woman) that as my dad's power of attorney, since he did suffer from dementia, I could, if I chose, fight his decision. I could stop his course of action. A single question floated to my lips.

"Why would I ever want to do that?"

A few days later, on February 25, 2010, surrounded by my mother and my wife, my father passed away. You'll notice I didn't mention myself. I was there, for sure. However, I was massively unprepared for what it would feel and look like. I remember going into the room before he died, and seeing him gasping with an unfocused stare in his eyes frightened me in ways I can't even begin to explain. My mother asked me to go to get my phone from the car to look up a Jewish prayer for her to say to him, and when I left the room, I never went back in. I held my daughter's car seat and stood in the hallway watching my mother and wife. I couldn't see him. I was afraid to.

I remember banging my forehead against the door placard with the room number on it as tears streamed down my face. I was wracked with sobs the likes of which I'd never felt or experienced before. My father was gone, at sixty-two years old, from complications arising from lifelong obesity. I'd never hear his laughter or voice again.

Two months later, on my 32nd birthday, I put his ashes into the waters of the Caribbean. My weight was already up more than thirty pounds since my race in 2009.

Nearly a year later, after struggling to get my business going and being successful at it, sadness would return as my maternal grandmother died in the same exact hospital.

In the meanwhile, my now ex wife and I started to struggle in a variety of ways. We are still friendly and good co-parents to this very day, so out of respect I won't detail the problems we had, except to say that neither of us was blameless. So we started weekly couples counseling, in addition to weekly personal counseling.

For two years we struggled through couples counseling before I came to the realization that I had given up hope entirely on our marriage ever getting better again. That moment—where I'd realized I had zero hope—was the turning point. That week in couples counseling, I told her that I no longer thought our marriage was viable.

We separated in 2014...amicably, albeit sadly. For our daughter's sake, however, we did everything we could to work together, and I'm proud to say we did a great job, to the point where we can (and will) even travel together on family trips from time to time. We have family dinners and meetings. Our daughter never has to wonder which side of the auditorium we're on when she has a school function, because we sit to-gether.

Through that period of time, I ended up with a new counselor personally. Dayna Pitsch (another dedication up front), who ended up being the single most skilled and insightful coun-selor I've ever worked with. She and I would address the fall-out from the divorce, issues I had with intimacy and attach-ment, struggles around dating, and more. All the while, my weight was steadily creeping upwards.

Flash forward (see? Told you I wasn't going to ask for sympa-thy? I was just setting the stage for some deeper understand-ing of where I was emotionally). By December of 2015 I'd reached a point where I knew change was necessary. I need-ed to try something new.

Something new as it turned out was a trip to Dr. Zeh. I had gotten to a point where my weight was high enough (approxi-mately 400 pounds) and my physical condition had deteriorat-ed enough that everyday things (walking around the grocery store, etc) were starting to hurt. And I was kind of tired of it. This moment, a meeting with Dr. Zeh on December 21st, 2015 ,was likely both my lowest point ever in this journey, but also at the same time the moment that saved my life.

CHAPTER 4

Coming to Terms – And Finding Hope

I knew my blood pressure was up, and I was already on medication for it. I knew my weight was up despite trying to get it under control. I knew I was running out of time. I was convinced that she was going to look at me and just throw her hands up and say "it's too late, we'll just give up on you now - better for you to die and just be done with it." I didn't want to die. I didn't want to give up. I had so much I was embarrassed about. But that's what I thought was about to happen. A slow march towards the grave.

In April of 2015, I'd registered for a runDisney half marathon in January, intending to lose the weight and be ready. I was going to get back onto the race course and recapture my passion for runDisney. But now, I couldn't exercise ten minutes without pain. I'd even had a bout of erectile dysfunction, which had *never* happened to me before. I realized I had too much on my plate personally and stopped dating altogether. I just couldn't handle it. I felt overwhelmed and lost. I felt like a failure, plain and simple. I felt hopeless. My weekly sessions with Dayna were devoted to managing the immediate stressors of the moment. But about two weeks before that doctor's appointment, sitting on Dayna's couch, I broke down. I told her about the physical difficulties I was having.

"For God's sake, Dayna, it hurts my back when I wipe my ass," I said to her through tears. I had no idea what could or should be done. But Dayna just sat with me through the tears and as they subsided she asked me why I didn't call my doctor to ask for help. I told her I was convinced she'd have given up on me by now. I had promised to lose the weight so many times in so many ways that surely there was no way she'd help me now that I was over 400 pounds. But Dayna encouraged me to make that appointment. She said it couldn't hurt.

Swallowing my fears and anxieties a little, I took the step. I picked up the phone and made an appointment to see Dr. Zeh.

At the appointment, I told her all of the things I'd told Dayna. I told her how I felt, what I feared, and what I knew she was going to do. Give up on me. I begged her for some sort of positive hopeful statement, but seemed convinced one couldn't possibly come. We'd discussed surgery in the past, and I'd always said no right off hand. I wouldn't have surgery, I was terrified of it. I could do it the old fashioned way. And a thousand other reasons. I wouldn't even listen to my doctor tell me to *consider* the possibility. But now I was desperate. I legitimately thought I was going to die. Soon.

"I'll do whatever you tell me to do. Want me to come in every week? I'll do that. Is it time for me to have the surgery? You told me to have it three years ago. I'll do it. Whatever you say." Already on that day I was on two blood pressure medications, an antidepressant, and a potassium supplement. My weekly counseling with Dayna had started nearly a year before, as I was having difficulty dealing with fallout from my separation and not having my daughter every day, not to mention the issues already discussed. I was, quite simply, a mess. I was at the bottom. This was my rock bottom moment. Rather than criticize or get angry, she shook her head and patted my hand as I started to tear up.

"No. It's not time for any of that. Your pressure is up again. But we're not even going to address that today. You don't have the strength right now to do anything to make progress. We're adding another antidepressant right now. Keep working with your counselor, and come back and see me in three weeks. In the meantime, you have an elliptical machine in your home, right? I want you to try to move a little every day. Even if it's only three minutes. Do something until it either hurts or stops being enjoyable. Work your way to ten minutes if you can. Just take baby steps. We'll keep working on it next month. But you're not hopeless. We're going to get through this." I sniffled and nodded. I wasn't a lost cause. There was hope.

After that day in Dr. Zeh's office, I felt supported in my quest moving forward. I had no idea what the quest was, but I felt like at least I wasn't alone. Dayna was immediately and completely supportive of the plan Dr. Zeh and I had come up with and we began discussing the possibilities moving forward. I admitted to her that I felt scared about the future, and embarrassed because I was scheduled to go to Walt Disney World in a few weeks (just after the first of the year) to run that runDisney half marathon. I'd committed to it in April and hadn't been able to get prepared. I was honestly considering just staying home. Dayna wouldn't have any of it.

"No. Your plane tickets are purchased and you're staying at that beautiful Animal Kingdom Lodge you mentioned. With the animals right outside your window. You're going. But I'm giving you permission to **not** feel bad about the race and to reframe this trip."

"What? Like some personal retreat?"

"Exactly."

And that's precisely what I did. I spent five days at the Animal Kingdom Lodge in Walt Disney World alone. I never left my room. I learned to meditate. I wrote and journaled. I slept. I pampered myself. And I just rested and focused on myself.

I should probably tell you that I hated being alone. I don't just mean on this retreat. I mean in general. Alone was never something I was any good at. Even at home, if I was alone too long, I'd find a way to engage someone or something or go out to be social (theatre, casinos, etc). And yet, at the Animal Kingdom Lodge, being alone felt not only okay, it felt necessary. It felt communal. Spiritual even. It felt like what I was meant to do. It gave me the moments of clarity and self care I needed to reach the single biggest decision I've ever made in my life.

It was in that room, with a giraffe outside my window, I decided that when I came home I was going to talk to my doctor about having weight loss surgery.

CHAPTER 5

As Safe as a Dance Party

It's amazing the way in which certain thoughts hit you at unexpected times. Something came up for me and it seemed
appropriate to talk about here a bit.

I have a thing about death. It's really annoying. And it's more
than the normal. I mean nobody I know of has ever been like
"yeah I'm great with death, bring it on, I'm looking forward to
it". But my issues with death get a little unusually neurotic.
Before I go any further, let me say this—I'm not going to place
faith or religion into this discussion. I have my own personal
faith, yes, but I'm also an educated skeptic. If you have
greater faith than me and this entire section seems unneces-
sary to you, I give you permission to skip it. I also envy that
level of faith. Although I have my own, I constantly wonder
what if I'm wrong? Which I guess means it's not really faith,
but rather hope, maybe?

Anyhow, death. The idea that everyone dies eventually isn't
my issue. I get that. Circle of Life and Simba and whatnot. The
fact that I might be wrong about what's after death is also not
the issue. Individual paradise, heaven, judgment, reincarna-
tion—all of these are viable and acceptable. My issue is noth-

ing. That's my issue. What if there's nothing? Now even that isn't really the issue. Here's where it gets a little neurotic.

I'm a type A control freak. I have to know the answers to things. I spend every day helping clients try to figure out all the possibilities and figuring out what they look like. The fact that I don't get to *know* what it's going to be like after death until I get there is hard enough, but the fact that there could be nothing causes my brain to go off the rails. Because as soon as I think about it, my brain tries to understand how it *feels* to *not exist.* Which is not only impossible, it'll make you crazy.

Add to that how much I love and adore my daughter and want her to have me for a long and happy life, and you start to understand why I'm writing about this today. See, last night, I was at the theatre, and all of a sudden, I was thinking about surgery and anesthesia. The fact that I could just...go out...and not wake up. I might never know and might never say goodbye to anyone. And it's something I'm doing voluntarily.

Then my rational brain kicks in and says that I do that every day I'm in a car. Take a risk that could kill me in an instant. But I've driven before. I've never had a chemical injected into my body that puts me to sleep. (Full disclosure: I did have a procedure at age 22 that required mild sedation, but I wasn't all the way out.)

This is apparently a common fear. I've done some basic research on the interwebs (and as you know if it's on there, it's true) and I'm happy to present to you some of my findings that are making me a little more comfortable. (*Disclaimer:* these numbers were what I found when I did the research for this at the time. These numbers may or may not be accurate now, then, or later. These numbers may or may not agree with your numbers or the numbers of your fellow scientists in the scientific community. Although if you have numbers of your own, you probably shouldn't be reading this section anyhow. Besides, I'm not presenting these to you as gospel fact. I'm presenting these to you as gospel 'How I learned to stop worrying and love the anesthesia'.)

In elective surgery, a healthy young to middle-aged patient has a risk of death due to complications from anesthesia of 1 in 250,000. When you include risk factors like age and severe illness the number increases to 1 in 60,000.

Here's some comparison death rates:

Hang Gliding: 1 in 560
Boxing: 1 in 2,200
Scuba Diving: 1 in 34.400
Canoeing: 1 in 10,000
Bicycling: 1 in 140,845
Mountain Hiking: 1 in 15,700
Mountain Hiking in Nepal: 1 in 167
Driving a Car: 1 in 6,700
Dance Parties: 1 in 100,000

The most important statistic I found however is this: people who are obese at 15+ years old are *THREE TIMES* more likely to die than those who aren't. So the only things safer are bicycling and having a dance party. Everything else is more dangerous than anesthesia. In fact, that became my new mantra when I worried about anesthesia: "As safe as a dance party."

Despite the coping tool, I knew I was still going to worry about it until surgery was done. But—*SPOILER ALERT*—you're reading this book. Even though I'm writing this portion before the surgery, I can't publish this until after the surgery and my weight loss success, which means I survived. So you will too. Okay? Good. No more freaking out.

CHAPTER 6

Survivor

I love watching television. I have lots of shows I enjoy, but the thing I enjoy most is a compelling narrative. I'm a storyteller at my core (lawyer, comedian, actor, writer, etc.) and love a story I can get lost in. One of life's most archetypical tales is the redemption story. This is mine, I believe. And here's how it relates to television.

About seven weeks before surgery, I went through biometric testing and body composition measurements. This was accomplished by sitting in something called the "BODPOD". I googled it and it looks a bit like a cryogenic chamber. *Maybe it really is. Maybe there's no surgery and they'll just freeze me for a few years until the weight comes off naturally. Doubtful, but who knows? I could actually end up MISSING the entire 2016 Presidential Election cycle, which would be a blessing in and of itself.*

In any event, the BODPOD apparently uses airflow to accomplish the measurements it needs. As a result, I had been asked to not wear any loose fitting clothing or anything with pockets or fabric breaks. The suggestion was bike or compression shorts. Yes, you read that right. They want a 400 lb.

man to squeeze himself into bike shorts. Before you spend any time visualizing it, ask yourself the question I had to ask. Where the hell do you *get* bike shorts that'll fit me?

With a little research online, I found a company that makes plus size men's compression and workout shorts. Precisely what I need. And they're branded. These are the "Official Workout Shorts of the *Biggest Loser*". Of all the television shows I watch, the *Biggest Loser* is one I've avoided. One of the reasons I avoid is it because I see myself in the contestants and don't have their success, which feeds into that cycle I mentioned earlier. Now I had to purchase an official *Biggest Loser* product. It was a bit disheartening. So I decided to off-set it with an empowering purchase as well.

You see, one of the shows I've recently become reacquainted (and mildly obsessed) with, is *Survivor*. This is a show that weaves interesting narratives through a challenging mental and physical competition. Plus Jeff Probst seems to never age, which is fascinating. I love watching a season and choosing my favorites and seeing how they evolve through the 39 days they spend together.

I'm a fan of choosing lofty goals and chasing after them. I've gone on record as saying that once this surgery is done and I'm getting thinner and stronger, I'll be working out, and one of my goals in my heart is to actually go compete on a season of *Survivor*. Imagine the guy who had bariatric surgery on *Survivor*! So after purchasing the official *Biggest Loser* shorts - symbolizing a show I never want to be on—I purchased an official *Survivor* Buff—symbolizing the show I'm going to be on someday. Also I plan on wearing my buff into every doctor's appointment, and even for surgery if they'll let me. Because whether or not *Survivor* ends up being something I'm able to do, I am in fact going to *survive* and thrive. That buff is so motivational. I could't wait to get it because the shorts had already arrived, and they were taunting me.

CHAPTER 7

Seminars - Hospitals - EVIVA

About six weeks before surgery, around late March 2016, I went to the pulmonologist's office...twice. I met with the psychologist (not Dayna, but the one from my surgical center), the fitness professional, and had my metabolic measurements and body composition tested by the MEDGEM and the BOD-POD, respectively. But alas, I'm getting ahead of myself. Let's get back to the January 2016 discussion, because although I may be approaching surgery in my personal timeline, I've just decided to have it in the timeline of this book. Wow! A time traveling book! And we're not even going 88 mph. I should also mention that this time hopping thing, which I've tried to keep at a minimum and clean up a little, is something my editor (and best friend) absolutely hates. But I think it's fun! So, back to January and my decision to have weight loss surgery.

Years before this decision was made, Dr. Zeh had suggested bariatric surgery to me several times as I'd struggled and struggled. I'd resisted. She kept encouraging me to at least *meet* with the Puget Sound Surgical Center, as their office (a private clinic) was right next door to hers. I still resisted. But now I was ready. After those three weeks on the new anti-depressant, I went in to see Dr. Zeh as planned. I had my questions ready from my personal retreat, and I was committed. I felt stronger.

"Okay, Doc. I'm ready to discuss surgery. Should I make an appointment next door?"

"Nope. I want you to go to the weight loss surgical seminar at our hospital."

A seminar? Wait. I wasn't planning on a seminar. Like a room full of people looking at me and thinking "ooooh, he needs surgery"? And what happened to Puget Sound Surgical? Dr. Zeh had full knowledge of the new program at their hospital and knew it was a robust program with education and aftercare. She thought it was essential that I had these tools for my success. It's a big name hospital that is very well respected in the area, so I wasn't upset by the referral, but I was a little surprised that next door was out of the running so quickly. I asked if it was okay that in addition to the seminar I did some research of my own on other locations. Of course she agreed.

Within two days I was registered for the Swedish Hospital Weight Loss Surgical Seminar. I had also discovered that Puget Sound Surgical had just rebranded themselves as "Eviva." From here on out, I'll refer to the first as Swedish and the second as Eviva, because, you know. Names. Anyhow, I decided to call Eviva for some information. It was a bit of an odd conversation. See, I knew I wanted surgery at this point, but what I didn't know was where. Or when. Or how. Or even what sort of surgery I wanted. Or could have.

"Eviva, how can I help you?"

"I'd like to get some information about surgery…" I said timidly.

"Sure. Let's get your contact information and Karin, our patient experience coordinator, will call you back soon."

Patient whatnow? Apparently Karin (who I hope is reading this because she's absolutely wonderful) was hired by Eviva for the sole purpose of calling potential patients and making them feel awesome and wonderful about Eviva and their services. She doesn't even work at their office. She works from home and is the liaison who schedules your surgical consult. She and I chatted for an hour about the different surgeries and why Eviva was where I wanted to do my surgery. It was a trifle sales pitchy, but then again I suppose it's supposed to be. I'm not going into details, as Eviva isn't paying me to write this book, but sufficed to say I was impressed by the personal level of care they provide and how enthusiastic Karin seemed about the process, not to mention their two year aftercare program. I happened to make this call the day before the Swedish seminar, and I told my best friend (editor - hi Jen!) that Swedish had to do a lot if they wanted to impress me as much as Eviva. They had an uphill battle.

The next night I drove to downtown Seattle to the Swedish Hospital for the weight loss seminar. I got there about 20 minutes early, as is my usual, and sat and watched while about twenty folks arrived. Each one looked nervous to be there and those who didn't come with a family member or friend glanced around from side to side as if they were waiting to rob a bank and wanted to make sure the coast was clear. Nobody spoke to anyone else and, in fact, nobody made eye contact. It was a nighttime seminar and we sat in the hallway and the over-whelming emotion I got from the group was shame. It didn't feel positive or hopeful even a little.

After an uncomfortable silent waiting area moment or two, the surgeon from the Swedish Weight Loss Clinic came and opened the conference room. Her name was Dr. Chen. She was about five feet tall and weighed approximately three-and-a-half pounds soaking wet. She was friendly, intelligent, and welcoming. She invited us all into the room and handed us informational folders with an insurance verification form paper clipped to the outside. It became obvious this was also going to be sales pitchy.

"As you're sitting down looking over the forms, we'll get start-ed soon, but if you'd like, we have some refreshments in the back." I could actually hear my stomach lurch. Nervously, my eyes started to dart around the room. Want to liven up a scared guy who's considering surgery and has a weight prob-lem? Tell me there's food.

"We have water, coffee, and tea." There was an audible sigh from the room. At least one guy groaned. Actually...both the sigh and groan came from *me*. I wanted to explain to this poor misinformed surgeon that what she had just offered me were not actually refreshments, but rather beverages. You do not tell me you have refreshments unless there's at least one food item on the table. I simply looked back at my materials and waited for Dr. Chen to tell me what I was there to hear.

Then the lecture began. Some interesting things came out of it, including the fact that obesity and being overweight are considered diseases by the FDA now. Apparently, it's no longer proper to say a person *is overweight* or *is obese*. Because the FDA recognizes it as a disease, we would now properly say a person *has obesity*. Like a person who HAS chickenpox. Although it doesn't absolve us of individual responsibility in our quests for physical fitness and health, it does help to alleviate some of the guilt. If I'm sick with a disease, then I'm not failing, I'm fighting. Surgery is a valid method of treating diseases, and so this is a surgical solution. Not a bad way to encapsulate it. Issue framing, not just for Karl Rove anymore.

Now we get to the sales portion of the seminar. Why the hospital program is better than private clinics. This is a paraphrase of their first attack on private clinics:

"Did you know that private clinics are owned by *doctors*? These people are doctors who cut corners to try to save money! They don't care about your well being as much as they do about their pocketbooks! They may do shorter surgeries, not take precautions, and won't let you stay overnight for observation. They'll operate on you in a back alley with a broken bottle and send you home still bleeding!"

Now I knew that doctors have an oath about not doing harm, but I'm also a business owner, and I had to wonder, did owning the business of surgery make you consider cost benefits?

I mean, even I look at different reams of paper before purchasing them to decide what's the most cost-effective. Did I want someone assessing cost effectiveness regarding the scalpels they were going to use to cut into me? I could barely think about that before she started in on her pitch for the hospital.

"What you want is a hospital, folks. I'm the head of the department, but I'm paid by the hospital, not you, so I'm not going to cut corners. I'm going to make sure you have the resources of an entire hospital at your disposal if you need it! Emergency? *Hospital.* Complication? *Hospital.* We have tons of anesthesiologists here, tons of doctors, nurses, beds , sheets, medicine, everything you need! Because *HOSPITAL.*"

That paraphrase pretty much summarizes her sales pitch. "Because hospital."

But the pitch is formulated on a miscalculation right off the bat. The assumption is that the doctors aren't interested in finances because they're employed by the hospital. Well guess what? The *hospital* is concerned with finances. Maybe even more so than a small clinic. I'll say this though: the idea of "what if there's a problem?" did stick in my mind. Maybe I did want a hospital.

So I called Karin at Eviva back. I specifically asked her about this concern. I wanted to know if hospital operating rooms were safer because they were surrounded by the rest of an entire hospital.

"Okay. Let's think about this, Jonathan. What's the most dangerous part of surgery?"

Wow. I hadn't considered that question.

"Knives?"

"Nope. Anesthesia."

Of course. That makes sense. Granted, it's as safe as a dance party. She continued.

"Anesthesia is weight based. Our doctors at our clinic only do bariatric surgery, and they have their own scrub teams, own nurses, and own anesthesiologists that they work with. All *those* people do is bariatric work. At a hospital, you'll get whoever is on call that day and they may not have as much bariatric experience."

Another really good point. That did it. Alright. I was ready to decide.

"Okay Karin. Let's do this. What's the next step."

"Let's get you set for your initial surgical consultation with your surgeon."

Now we were getting somewhere. I'd made a bold decision and was ready to accept that decision and whatever it meant moving forward. Granted, I had no idea what it actually meant.

I was first given an option of a younger doctor at their practice who Karin didn't know much about. Hopefully I didn't offend her by asking what my other options were.

Second option. A doctor who had been with their practice for fifteen years and was quite good with his surgical technique. However, Karin described his "demeanor" as occasionally blunt. My optimism was sinking a little. I was nervous, and needed someone I could connect with and who made me feel safe. I timidly asked if there was another option.

"Well look at that! I can get you in to see Dr. Landerholm. He's one of our founders. He's been doing this since the beginning. His work is flawless and he had a focus originally on plastics. You probably won't even have too noticeable of a scar."

"What about his personality?" I was going to have to deal with this surgeon not only through the surgery but for the two year aftercare program too. I wanted someone I could have faith in.

"Honestly? You can't tell him I told you this, okay?" I assured Karin I wouldn't tell him, but since I'm writing this now, I assume Karin doesn't mind.

"He's so nice and charismatic we have a nickname for him. We call him Doctor Smooth Jazz."

Now *that* was my guy.

CHAPTER 8

Doctor Smooth Jazz

We set my surgical consult for the next week. I informed Dr. Zeh, who was immediately on board and knew Dr. Landerholm well. Dayna was ecstatic that I'd made such a decision. But there was still a hard conversation left to have. I had to tell my mother I was having surgery. My mother, who is a retired RN, asked to come with me. Actually, "asked" really isn't the right word. Demanded is more like it. She's tough on medical professionals and anytime she sees one, she is full of appropriate questions and terminology. She was going to grill this poor Doctor, I was sure of it. But I guessed I could use the backup and maybe someone to explain the bigger words to me. After all, I'm only a lawyer.

This is a great time to discuss insurance. In Washington State, *some* private group insurances cover this surgery. But as a sole legal practitioner, I have an individual plan. Not one individual plan covers this surgery. The overall cost of the surgery out of pocket is $21,000. There are time payment loans available, but rather than that, in what amounted to the greatest birthday present ever (my birthday is April 17th- just a few weeks before my surgical date), my mother simply offered to cover the cost. I'm a single dad paying spousal support and struggling with a small law practice. I couldn't be doing this without her support both emotionally and financially. So I'll just say thanks, Mom. I love you. (If you were paying attention, she's the Kay in the dedication at the beginning of the book).

As I said, my mom is one of those nurses who tells everyone she's a nurse and isn't afraid to get in the conversation about anything medical. We went to my initial consultation and I was prepared for her to pepper Dr. Smooth Jazz with questions.

I'd already decided that the surgery in question was going to be Gastric Sleeve surgery. There are currently three major types of bariatric (weight loss surgery) that are prevalent in America. Here's my understanding of the three and why I chose what I chose.

1) Lap Band Surgery: This is where they take essentially a hard rubber hair tie and wind it around the top of your stomach, so it limits the amount of food you can have. It was popular for awhile because it's reversible. Patients who have it tend to lose the least weight, and are signing themselves up for years of further surgeries because the band needs to be adjusted frequently. That being said, unlike Gastric Bypass, there are fewer digestive side effects.

2) Gastric Bypass Surgery: Here they reroute your intestinal tract around your stomach entirely. Think of it as a highway bypass loop around a major city. No traffic in or out of the city, just fast travel around it. You're limited in quantity, and in terms of what you can eat, because apparently the stomach is an important part

of the digestive process. Without it in the loop, there's limits to what you can eat. Patients who have this surgery tend to lose the most weight, but it's also the most extreme surgery.

3) Gastric Sleeve Surgery (Goldilocks surgery): Here they just cut out 85% of your stomach. That's all. Actually the 85% they remove (the fundus for you anatomy geeks out there) is really not all that important, and has the fun side effect of being one of the only places in the human body that produces the hormone that tells your brain you're hungry. SCORE! This surgery generally has patients who lose about 2-3% *less* weight than with the bypass, but have much fewer complications, because you still have a stomach. This is now the preferred "gold standard" surgery for weight loss. We have a winner!

I was told about several consultations I needed before surgery. I also told him that I wanted to have surgery May 4th. He penciled it in and we started scheduling consultations.

Pulmonology: Likely because of my size and weight and the fact that I had sleep apnea, this was essential. Actually I told Dr. Landerholm that I had never been diagnosed with sleep apnea, but he simply said he didn't care. I had it. He wanted it formally diagnosed and treated. Sleep apnea is when your airway closes when you're sleeping for a second or two. Postop I would be on pain medications that would suppress my breathing already and this could result in the unfortunate outcome of me going to sleep and waking up dead. This seemed like a reasonable thing to look into.

Mental Health: I had to be cleared by the Eviva psychologist to have surgery. This is apparently required by the Federal Government because of the permanent and irreversible nature of the surgery I was having. I have to be okay with and understand the fact that a part of me was coming out and wouldn't ever go back in. Compare this to gastric bypass and/ or lapband surgery, both of which can be reversed.

Biometrics: This is the aforementioned BODPOD. It gives us a baseline to measure success as we go.

Nutrition and Exercise: This would prepare me both pre and post op for how my life was going to change and what I needed to give up and begin doing.

The consultation lasted about an hour and a half. My mother asked not one single question and said almost no words at all. I was floored. I assumed she wasn't asking questions because she was satisfied. After scheduling my appointments, we walked out and I decided to ask her. Her response was rather unexpected.

"I'll tell you this, Jonathan. That is one *good looking surgeon*. And he had no wedding ring on."

Doctor Smooth Jazz indeed.

CHAPTER 9

To Sleep Perchance to Breathe

My pulmonologist appointment was set for about a week later. I knew I was going to have to do a sleep study. Sleeping hadn't been good. I snored. I dozed off around 5pm many days. I was sure I had apnea. My ex wife had apnea too. She went through a sleep study where she stayed away a night and had things attached to her head and whatnot. She came back with a huge bulky loud machine that she could never get used to. I assumed I'd have the same struggles. I was wrong. I had entirely different struggles.

When I arrived at the pulmonologist's office, I was a bit early. They were happy to see me and took me into the back room to meet with the technician. She measured my neck and chest and took some readings of breathing and whatnot. Then she told me she'd be back and would let the doctor know I was ready. They would come and get me when they were ready for me.

My appointment time came. And went. The door to the room I was in was closed. I could hear voices outside the door, including one that I assumed belonged to the doctor. They were talking about how one of their appointments no-showed and they could likely break for lunch early. Early like right at that moment. I was about to say something when the technician came in to get her purse.

"Oh! I forgot you were back here!"

Sounds about right. Hard to miss when I'm seen, hard to remember when I'm not. So they ushered me into the doctor's office. He was rather apologetic about me being...well...forgotten. He asked why I was there.

"Surgical clearance. Everyone says I have apnea."

"Nice of them to diagnose you for me. I'll leave it to my own judgment, thank you."

Okay. This guy was definitely *not* smooth jazz. After talking to him for awhile though he clearly knew his stuff. He's an apnea sufferer too. So he's coming at this from an angle where he could clearly understand it. He reiterated to me that treating apnea was really critical in making sure that I didn't, you know, die, in my post operative recovery. Made sense to me. But he wasn't sure I had apnea.

"So we'll do a sleep study."

"Okay doc. When do I come in for it?"

"Nope. You'll do it at home. Tonight."

Say what? At home? Sure enough there was an at-home sleep study machine they were able to give me. I had to pick what time I'd fall asleep that night and then strap myself to two, hard, metal boxes, one around my belly button, one around my chest. I'd also be wearing a a finger monitor and a nasal canula to measure my exhalation. These machines would measure my heart and breathing rate as well as my pulse oxygen. Trying the thing on at the office felt a bit like Darth Vader getting suited up. Minus the James Earl Jones.

I bagged it up and headed home. When I wore it later that night I was bare chested, and when I put on the nasal canula I decided to take a look at myself in the mirror to see what I looked like, expecting Darth Vader, or at least some sort of super hero. I instantly started tearing up.

You see, as I've mentioned, my father was my idol. My hero really. In addition to what I've already discussed, he also suffered from, yes—sleep apnea. Severe apnea. He had what is called a biPap machine. Late in his life, he was on oxygen permanently for that vascular dementia I mentioned because his pulse oxygen would drop to the point where his brain wouldn't function properly and he'd get confused. He had a constant nasal canula for the last several months of his life.

Looking in that mirror seeing myself with a canula on and being shirtless and overweight was almost too much to handle. I was not willing to consider myself dying this way. I was not willing to wear a canula any longer than I had to. I was going to do this study and this surgery and really succeed. I was getting rid of this canula as soon as I possibly could. If not sooner.

Then I tried laying down. With metal boxes on me. It was uncomfortable. I slept in fits. When I woke up one of the cords had disconnected from the main box. Crap. I was going to have to re-do this thing wasn't I?

Sure enough when I returned the machine to the home sleep study unit they told me almost immediately I'd have to rerun it that night. This time they taped the hell out of the unit, including the wires and whatnot and that night I tried again. When I awoke I was still connected. Eureka! I dropped off the unit and waited my two days for my follow up appointment.

I was diagnosed with average (moderate) sleep apnea. They gave me a CPAP machine and showed me a mask to use with it. So since you may not know what a CPAP is, it's a machine that hooks to a mask that covers your nose (or in my case, rests, pillow-like, under the nose) and blows air into your nostrils all night long so that if you stop breathing (apnea) air is forced in so you don't die. (As an aside, I was really impressed with just how much these folks were into the idea of me not dying.)

It also allows you to get a better night's sleep overall by allowing you to keep sleeping deeply when you'd normally wake a smidge. The masks they showed me ranged from one that covered your entire nose, to nasal pillows that go inside your nose, to a pillow that goes under the nose with one big hole for the air. That's the one I selected. The mask was actually called the "Dream Mask", which sounded lovely. I'll say it took a few days to get used to, but as a stomach sleeper, I think I wasn't helping myself out at all. I had to give up a ton of things

I loved. I'd be damned if I was going to give up tummy sleeping!

CHAPTER 10

Fitness - Eating - Psych

Now that the Apnea was under control, I was off to Eviva's main facility where I was to meet with biometrics, exercise, nutrition, and mental health. Checking off all in one day was going to make life a lot easier. I really liked the efficiency of that part of the process.

First up after checking in was biometric measurements. We've already discussed my *Biggest Loser* compression shorts, which I put on for this portion of the day. I was then handed the MedGem, which looked a lot like a portable breath testing device. (I know a lot about those as I'm a DUI attorney when I'm not writing books and losing weight and acting and winning Survivor). I had to hold it in my mouth for nine minutes. Why nine and not ten or eight? I have no idea. I asked, and received a shrug as my answer. But I had to hold it in my mouth and breath normally. This apparently told them something about my basal metabolic rates and breathing patterns, or gave them the opportunity to look at me through a window and giggle.

After that, it was time to get into the BODPOD. When I entered the room and saw it for the first time, I immediately thought of every science fiction movie I've ever seen. The Google image search I did was completely accurate and it did, in fact, look like a cryo-sleeping chamber. I sat in it, and it was sealed airtight. There was air inside, and as it moved and displaced, it measured my body mass. 45 seconds later I had a printout and was out of the BODPOD. So much for cryogenically missing the surgery entirely.

I was told to sit there and wait for Dameon, my fitness advisor. I did so and within a few minutes, a rock solid, bald man walked in and shook my hand with the tightest grip I've ever felt. This guy was lean and thin, and had to be in the negative percentages of body fat. He sat down and asked a little about my fitness experience. I told him about having competed in seven half marathons in the past and my goal being to get back out there someday. I have an elliptical and treadmill in my home. I have my own set of free weights and have loved lifting in the past. I told him I wanted to be strong enough to get onto Survivor and get out there for another runDisney event. I expected him to want to do a fitness evaluation with me and determine where I was starting from so we had a baseline. Nope.

"Well you've got a good plan, and I'm here to help you. You know what you're doing and anytime you want to come and workout here, let me know. We have walking groups and whatnot too!"

According to another employee, Dameon was a very different fitness advisor who is hardcore in terms of workouts, but didn't mince words or want to put you through needless tests and education if you already knew what you were doing.

"In the meantime, man, just start moving more." I told him my back and legs tended to hurt. "Yep. And as you move more they'll hurt less."

Fair enough. Fitness over, time to see nutrition.

I knew that two weeks before surgery I would begin my "official" pre-op diet. I say "official" because I started about two weeks before that. My doctor wanted me to lose about ten pounds prior to surgery in addition to the pre-op diet, so I started early. The pre-op diet is a liver shrinking diet so that the "operating theatre" has more room for my doctor to do his thing, as the stomach is right next to the liver. How do you shrink your liver, you ask? Good question. Take in no more than 40g of carbs per day and limit your caloric intake to around 1600 per day. You might be surprised to know that *after* the surgery I likely wouldn't have to limit carbs. I'll explain.

My nutrition appointment simply gave me a preview of what life would be like after the surgery. Of primary import after the surgery is preserving the lean muscle mass on your body because it burns fat. Apparently for someone in my size and shape range, to do so you need 60-80 grams of protein per day. But not me. Oh no. My BODPOD readings were so unusually high in lean mass that I was told I would literally not be able to consume enough protein to maintain it. But it's about making sure you take in enough protein. That's it.

It was time to discuss goal setting and my preoperative diet. We wrote down some things. We also identified some things to eliminate from my world entirely. Alcohol, which I didn't drink, so no problem. Minimize caffeine...I might have a coffee from time to time. Carbonated beverages.

HOLD UP. What?!?

Yes. No carbonation. It can cause massive discomfort and other problems. The nutritionist's eyes nearly bulged when I told her I could polish off 3 two liters of Diet Coke *every day.* I was going to have to give it up. Which I've done before. I've switched to flavored carbonated water. Oops. No carbonation. Seltzer? Nope.

Crystal light is my new friend. No carbs. Five calories. No carbonation. Not as boring as plain water. Lots of flavors.

So we wrote down goals. Minimize carbs. Cut out carbonated beverages. Start moving more. Download apps to help with all this. (There are **tons. M**y favorite happens to be MyFitness-Pal.) We discussed supplementation and protein drinks and whatnot. Although it was very vague and quiet on the post op stuff, it was quite specific on the pre op stuff. Apparently I'd see the dietician after my preoperative appointment to discuss post op.

I was escorted from nutrition upstairs to mental health, which is a FDA required session before anyone has this type of surgery. The therapist had to discuss with me that I would need support both before and after. He had to make sure I understood how to get help should I need it. But the most interesting part of that meeting, as I mentioned, was when the therapist had to confirm that I understood the "permanent and irreversible nature" of my surgery.

Well, yeah. I get it doc.

"But do you? They are removing a part of your body. It will be outside you. You can't have it back."

The only response I could think of was more honest than I was expecting.

"Thank god. Take it." Maybe I was actually starting to look forward to this process. Maybe even be, dare I say it, *excited* about the prospect.

"Okay. You understand. Sign here."

Apparently I was sane enough to have the surgery. Well I'm glad someone acknowledged my sanity.

CHAPTER 11

Disclosures – i.e. – You Might Die

The CPAP machine had its share of problems when I started. The masks I tried would slip off my head at night, so finding the right mask with the right fit was a process. Regardless, I was able to figure it out with trial and error. It would still slip off sometimes, but less often and I was learning to live with it.

Time with the CPAP passed and I suddenly found myself face to face with my preoperative appointment. I had to bring my "support person" with me for these meetings, which meant my best friend and editor extraordinaire, Jen (Sup Jen?!). Two days before my preoperative appointment I was called in by the anesthesiologists asking me to come in to have them check on me because I was "so tall". At least, that's what the receptionists had told me. That seemed odd. I'm six foot two. Not grossly over tall by any means. Apparently what they wanted to do was make sure I wasn't so big that we'd have to do the surgery in the hospital instead of the outpatient clinic. Thankfully I wasn't. I thought the "too tall" thing was kind of strange. So did the anesthesiologist.

"I told them I wanted to evaluate you because of your size. They assumed height. Jeez, it's not like we *only* do bariatric surgery or anything here!" Sarcasm, while appreciated, did not help my mindset when it was about the intelligence of the people scheduling my surgery. As long as the preop appointments went without a hitch, things would be fine.

They asked me to arrive about 30 minutes early for the appointment. Which I did, because I was hyper about making sure everything went right, because I was afraid of it all. So arrive early, I did, only to find out that I was at the wrong location. Preop day was a really crazy amount of running around from place to place. But I somehow managed to see everyone that I needed to.

When I saw the surgeon (not Dr. Smooth Jazz, as he was out) we went through a list of "disclosures" and "risk forms." Basically I signed about seventeen thousand things saying that I totally understand that I could die from this surgery and complications from it. Then we discussed the risks in full as well as what to expect after the surgery medically.

Yes. I understood I might have died. I understood I might have fallen asleep and not woken up. I understood that a thousand things could go wrong before, during, and after the surgery and that any one of them could kill me. But the worst part wasn't understanding, it was having to put my name down on it. I had to write my acceptance of the risks. As if it were okay to kill me!

I found out we were stopping two of my blood pressure medications. When I asked why we were going to do that I was shocked to find out that the surgery often helps reduce blood pressure all on its own and that if we kept the medication in place, I could bottom out which would also be bad. In case you're wondering, by bottoming out, what they meant was kill me.

But the surgery could literally cure my hypertension right off the bat. I knew it would help, but not to the point where we'd be removing medications right away. I'd be monitoring my pressure at home and seeing how it went. Which seemed exciting, but also alien. I'd been on blood pressure medications for literally years. When I went off them I felt like crap. But now they were making me willingly stop.

Every time I asked a question like this, however, the surgeon (and later Dr. Smooth Jazz himself) would just get a knowing little smirky smile and a glimmer in their eye, as if to say "oh you poor misinformed soul, just you wait until I make you anew." It was confidence inspiring. Far more than the schedulers who couldn't seem to get me to the right place on the right day!

I was also told to get up and walk around the room every hour or so. I was really struggling to understand the full impact of the exhaustion and pain I was going to be feeling. I was unprepared and unaware. I just didn't know. I did know they prescribed anti nausea medicine and some pretty hefty pain killers for me. So hey, there was that.

We discussed fevers, infections, rips, tears, vomiting, and everything in between. Oh yeah…and death too. Did I mention death? Because they sure as hell did. It was quite a lovely conversation. But us lawyers caused all this ruckus so I only have myself to blame, I suppose. Thanks law school!

Then it was off to nutrition to discuss the preoperative diet, and more importantly the post-operative diet! Finally I'd learn what this was all going to be. After the surgery my stomach would be swollen and healing for days. My body would apparently be learning to accept food and drink again, like from scratch. I'd be just relearning everything. To accommodate that, here's what the first two weeks would look like—and lest we forget: I would be trying to get in 80+ grams of protein a day doing this.

Two days post op: Clear liquids only. Broths and whatnot. According to the nutritionist, due to the swelling in the stomach a drink of eight ounces should take me about two hours to finish. Before surgery I could do it in two large gulps.

Seven days after that: Pure liquids—creams and soups, etc.

Seven days after that: Purees—the baby food diet.

After that: Back to normal food. But get this, my portion size moving forward would be about 3/4 of a cup. Total. Per meal. Period. And not only was that supposed to fully satisfy me— any more and I'd get sick.

To make sure I got the nutrients I needed, I was now going to be on a very regimented supplementation regime including multivitamins, B12, and calcium several times daily.

Which prompted me to ask about nutrition on *Survivor,* because we all know that's where I was headed, at least in my brain. After a slight negative response (there's just no way without proper nutrition...we just can't....or can we?), I got the nutritionist on my side.

"Well we could give you a massive B12 shot before you go...."

Yes. We were going to do this. Surgery. Health. *Survivor.* A mere ten days away. What a journey I had to look forward to! If I could avoid the whole dying part.

CHAPTER 12

Meatsticks

When I was done with the nutritionist, she showed me to the store they had set up. I was able to buy my chewable vitamins, and several other products. Now let's be clear about the store itself. I say store because there were shelves and you could buy stuff off the shelves. But the size of this store was impressive. Impressively small. Consider your average coat closet. Now jam it with shelves and bariatric products. That was it. Maybe half that size. A fraction of half that size. Think of a portion of a fraction of that size and then take a sliver. Then call it a store.

I bought my vitamins. I also bought some Isopure tea, a clear liquid with 40 grams of protein per bottle, and nothing else really. Not a bad supplement for my liquid days, I figured. I had no idea how it'd taste, but I was pretty sure I wouldn't care.

I bought some soups for the soup days, and some OsTrim meat sticks. Yes, I said meat sticks. Stop giggling. Children. They're quite yummy and only have 2g of carbs, and lots of protein in a 90 calorie package. Useful on my preoperative diet.

Then I joined the official EVIVA Facebook group. What an amazing group of people I found there. It's an invite only group and I simply made a post to introduce myself. The range of wonderful responses I got almost immediately was overwhelming. Here's a sample:

"Welcome!! Sending you good surgery vibes..."

"You are going to love the new you!!"

"Welcome to the most wonderful journey!"

"You'll need a new wardrobe sooner than you think."

"Welcome, Jonathan! It's an amazing journey and the best decision I've ever made!"

"Welcome to the loser's lounge!"

"Get ready to be a new person and feel like even more of a hottie!"

That last one made me chuckle. I wondered what the hell I'd feel like as a "hottie". Hottie was never a word I'd heard used to describe me at all before. The idea that the outside packaging could more easily reflect the energy and confidence I'd start feeling inside was a really new frontier. What would that feel like? When? How would I know? These people seemed to have been where I was, and were a welcoming and insightful group of people who wanted nothing more than to help me through this. So I started asking them for ideas to help me survive...well...*Survivor.* They're still working on it with me as of this writing. We'll get there together and it'll be great.

Speaking of surgery prep, my preop diet was going great. Often for breakfast I would have a lovely veggie omelette with some chorizo and a few small strips of extra crispy bacon, which was always delish. I'd also ordered some amazing protein products from Amazon to help out: shakes, bars, and more. Here's a tip for you if you're looking for protein products—try different brands. Things taste differently depending on which brand you choose, and not all brands are created equal. For instance, Muscle Milk light shakes have a really weird bitter aftertaste, while Pure Protein shakes are quite nice. Premier Protein (which is usually available at Costco) are hands down the best, agreed by most, not sure why. But find what works for you, and don't overstock until you know what you like. I say this as someone who's actually thrown out four boxes of rather expensive protein bars I bought because the flavor "birthday cake batter explosion" sounded amazing, but when I bit into the first one, after nearly breaking a tooth, I realized that the birthday cake in question was clearly made for Shrek out of dung beetles and mud.

You know, at this point I was just about a week away from the big surgery day and with the one week countdown happening, I wasn't quite as nervous as I thought I'd be. I was just starting to get plain old excited. And you, dear reader, should be too, because the "backstory" is all done now. Now I'll be writing this story to you in real time. What I'm writing will be about now, now. Then is past and soon is coming, but now we're at now.

Gotta love Mel Brooks.

CHAPTER 13

Prepping - Shaving - Navels - and Sleepy Time

I shaved my head. Completely. For the first time in my life. I was surprised that I liked how it looked. Made me look tougher, I think. Especially if I put on sunglasses and crossed my arms. Why did I shave my head? Apparently one of the occasional side effects of this surgery for men is hair loss. Since my hair was already thinning I decided to just head it off at the pass and do it myself.

Two days prior to surgery, in the morning, my phone rang. It was Jillian from EVIVA. She wanted to go through some last minute instructions for me and tell me when my surgery was scheduled. Apparently my surgery was scheduled for 2:15pm, and I was to arrive at 1:00pm wearing comfortable, loose fitting clothing and any overnight items I might want to have with me.

"I recommend you bring entertainment or electronic devices because we don't have TVs but we do have free Wi-Fi." Wow we've come a long way, haven't we?

I had to stop certain medications and was not allowed to eat after 6:00pm the night before, nor was I allowed to drink after 7:00am the day of surgery. But then she gave me an instruction that puzzled me a little bit.

"Also we ask you please clean your belly button before surgery."

Clean my belly button? Why? Are we doing belly button pictures? Is it going to be shown off somehow?

So I used my trusty computer and dug a little (hehe—belly button humor). Apparently with laparoscopic surgeries often they use the navel for an incision site and they want you to pre-clean it so you avoid infections and complications. So okay...a good shower with a navel cleaning it would be.

Nerves. Friends who knew I was having the surgery were starting to ask me if I was nervous. What's funny is that every time they asked, I got *more* freaking nervous. I was honestly scared. I mean, I knew the odds (as safe as a dance party) and that many people much less healthy than I have survived surgery with no problems. But what if I went to sleep on anesthesia and didn't wake back up? What about saying goodbye to people? Seeing my daughter? Everything! Honestly that's the thing that scared me. I wasn't scared of the cuts or the healing or the aftercare process. I was just scared that I wouldn't wake back up.

Which I knew, of course, was silly. Breathing and counting to five calmed me down and I'd quickly be back in excitement mode for the new life awaiting me.

But I figured you might be scared too. So I'd say something.

All at once, the moment was here. It was May the Fourth (be with me) and I hadn't eaten since 6:00pm the night before. No liquids since midnight. They'd actually called me in *early* because they were ahead of schedule. Imagine a doctor's office being ahead of schedule.

I was sitting in my preoperative suite talking to my preoperative nurse, Jeruschia, who was making me smile and laugh. This despite having signed about seventeen forms that all said "I understand the surgery, what will happen, and the fact that I might die." My belly button was cleaned and I was ready for this to happen. I'd lost fifteen pounds on the preoperative diet. I weighed in at 390 pounds the day of surgery.

My personal support team, consisting of my mother and my best friend, Jennifer, (who is also my editor, as I've mentioned—HI AGAIN, JEN!) were there with me in the preoperative suite helping me relax. I only asked for two things. First, I wanted them to stay with me and keep my brain occupied beforehand. Secondly, I did not want to wake up alone. I was promised both.

Now, before the surgery would begin, the anesthesiologist came in to tell me a bit more about what to expect. I was pretty sure I knew how this was going to go, because I'd seen TV and movies and, of course, knew what to expect.

"So the first thing we'll do is put a mask on you."

"For the gas?"

"No. We don't do gas. It's oxygen. See, once you're out, you stop breathing. I have to put three tubes into your throat. One for breathing, one to inflate your abdomen with carbon dioxide, and one for the camera so they can see. When you stop breathing, bad things happen, so I want to get you to 100% oxygen before I put you out, so you don't die while I'm tubing you."

Gulp.

"Okay. Makes sense." My heart rate jumped.

"Next, I'm going to tell you…" I knew this one, so I interrupted.

"To count backwards!"

"No. We don't do that. I'm going to tell you to think of a pleasant thought. See, I don't know if you're going to dream or not while you're under, but if you are dreaming, I want it to be something pleasant. So when I tell you to think of something pleasant, that's your cue that it's just about sleepy time."

Something about him calling it "sleepy time" made it seem less like the whole "not breathing might die" thing, so I was okay with it.

Almost as soon as the conversation was over, my nurse was there and told me it was time. I looked around the suite for my wheelchair or gurney. Nope. We were walking to the surgical suite. *WALKING.* Like on the way down *The Green Mile.*

We walked down a hallway and turned a corner into the operating room. There was the operating table, complete with arm board and straps. Essentially a lethal injection table. I felt my heart thumping in my chest like a bass drum.

"Just hop up on the table and scoot down. We'll get you secured."

I lay down on the table and my breathing was elevated as was my blood pressure. I could feel the pulsing in my head. I was starting to freak out. Before I had a chance to think, here came the mask.

"Just breath deeply for me."

Now my brain took over.

Hey. You know what, man? We've lost fifteen pounds through the preoperative diet. That's not so bad. It was manageable. Maybe we just keep doing that. Yeah. Let's do that. We'll just stay on the preoperative diet and go home. Maybe we just cancel this thing.

"Okay, time to think of something pleasant."

Oh shit.

Next thing I remember, I was sitting in a chair in the dark in my preoperative suite, barely aware of anything, except for one really important fact. I was alive.

Alone and Farting Your Cares Away

I was also alone.

I was awake and in my suite, fading in and out of a cloudy pain medication haze. It was dark outside, and my surgery had been in the early afternoon. Clearly things had changed. I was sore as hell on my abdomen, but I had work to do, apparently. I spoke a few words, and I'll be honest, I'm not sure what they really were, but they were enough to get the attention of my night nurses, Kayla and Lisa.

Apparently I hadn't been alone the whole evening. Jen and my mother had stayed, and according to Kayla and Lisa, had entire conversations with me before leaving. I had absolutely no memory of this. I've also come to learn afterwards that I demanded Jen call my ex-wife and talk to her because I'd promised my daughter I'd call when I was awake. Jen felt a little weird about that as she'd never even met my ex-wife at this point, but apparently I insisted. I have zero memory of this happening, but in my imagined reality it was pretty funny to me at the time. Apparently, even though I wasn't *quite* awake yet, my mother had wanted to go home and on the way asked if she could stop and have some dinner, so Jen obliged. Then Jen came back to see me for the aforementioned call to my daughter. Although I was "awake" during this period of time, I have zero actual memory (maybe a fuzzy moment or two) of it.

Kayla and Lisa offered me more meds and lots of fluids. Water, and then some hot broth which felt exquisite going down my throat. I had expected my abdomen to hurt, for Pete's sake; I had six separate cuts in it. I didn't expect my throat to be killing me from three tubes, though.

Still, I had no idea what pain was yet. Because shortly thereafter, Lisa and Kayla wanted me to walk to the end of the hall. They also wanted me to try to pee. Both of these things were slow going, painful, and rather humorous as I was plodding a little step at a time down the hallway with my butt hanging out of my gown.

This is a moment where I'd like to acknowledge another person who was instrumental in my journey. Keith is a sixty-plus year old man who had his sleeve surgery the same day and was in the suite next to mine. We'd pass each other as we walked the halls, and later connected via Facebook in the Eviva Facebook group. But this was the first moment I laid eyes on my #sleevebrother. So hey, Keith!

Each walk also involved coughing and deep breathing. This apparently is designed to do two things. Thing one: clear the lungs and avoid pneumonia. Thing two: *hurt like hell*. Every time I coughed, I felt my abdominal muscles (which had been literally *cut open*) reminding me that they'd been literally *cut open*.

At 4:00am that morning I was discharged and headed home with Jen, who was my "support person". She was required to stay with me 48 hours after surgery to make sure I walked, coughed, and I guess, didn't die or anything. Since I'm here and writing this, and she's editing it, clearly she did her job well. So thanks again, Jen!

The first day home was kind of a blur of sleepiness and being encouraged to get up and walk around and also to drink even more fluids. Sip sip sip. If I sipped too much, or gulped in any air, or even swallowed any air, my esophagus would tell me. With pain. Like an elephant sitting on my chest. So I had to relearn how to sip things.

And oh what wonderful things I could sip! Here's a list of what I consumed in the first three days of being home (72 hours):

1. 11 ounce Crystal Light drinks
2. Two 20 ounce bottles of Isopure Protein Tea
3. Two 11 ounce Pure Protein Shakes
4. Three four ounce cups of broth

For my first "dinner" meal I decided to have yogurt, which you can't really sip, but you can take small bites. Because too much and there's that elephant. Although he hangs around because of the bloating too.

Yes, I said bloating. Remember that Carbon Dioxide I mentioned earlier? Yep, my abdominal cavity was massively tight and full. Burping and hiccuping (which I did a lot of) hurt…a lot. But then all of a sudden it happened. It was glorious.

I farted. Many times. And every time it felt wonderful. Over and over.

Jen commented that they had no smell for as much as I'm farting.

"Because there's nothing to digest—no methane in there, Jen. Just CO2. Hell, if I had potted plants in here they'd perk up every time I fart!"

And before you tell me that writing about gas is uncouth, you wait until *you* are three days post op and the Gas-X strips aren't quite alleviating the pain. You'll fart. Trust me. And you'll love every second of it.

CHAPTER 15

One Week Checkup - Baby Food - and Dumping

After seven days, I had my one week post op check with Dr. Smooth Jazz himself. First we weighed in and I was down to 381.2 meaning I'd lost 8.8 pounds in the week after surgery. Not bad. Then we checked my wounds, which looked good, and discussed moving forward. Nine days post op would be a big day. I would be transitioning from a pure liquid diet to purees. Wow.

I also learned things I hadn't really known before. The preoperative diet that they'd put me on wasn't actually to lose weight. The low carb diet was designed to shrink my liver, because the liver is what sits on top of the stomach, which is an important thing for them to reach. Well, lo and behold, apparently my liver hadn't shrunk as much as they'd have liked to see pre-op, and for a few minutes during the beginning of the surgery, Dr. Smooth Jazz couldn't get a good view of what he needed to see. They actually considered closing me up and doing the surgery another day. I would have been furious. Thankfully he was a very skilled doctor and managed to do it all. No worries—surgery done. Which begs the question: If it was a no harm, no foul situation, why even bother to tell me?

So I advanced to purees, which includes things like cottage cheese, ricotta cheese, smoothies, mashed potatoes, and more. All of course in tiny quantities (starting at 1/4 cup per meal) and needing to be high protein. Did you know they make unflavored protein powder you can add to things like potatoes? Apparently that's a thing. Except it's not unflavored. When you add it to potatoes it makes them taste vaguely like dirty potatoes. I wasn't a fan. However, ricotta mixed with a packet of Splenda and a teaspoon of vanilla extract made me feel like I was eating the filling out of a cannoli. Now we're talking!

The first few days home and alone after Jen left gave me a lot of time to think about things, and it brought up some significant issues for us to discuss. Many of us (myself included) battle with negative emotions and depression. Isolation can heighten that at times. I found my mind wandering to sad and darker thoughts quite often during those few days. Just looking over at my board games and longing to have someone to play something with at that very moment. This could have been related to me being a single dad where I only have my daughter half time, and since I was recovering from surgery, not being able to see her as long as I would normally. This could have been related to many of my friends being married with kids and as such having such limited schedules. It could even just have been because I took a week off from my improv classes to heal.

Regardless. Emotions happen to us all. And they can and will happen to you during this process. I'm here to tell you that it's okay to just feel them. Experience the emotion. Learn from it. See what it feels like. You are getting to learn about a brand new you that is emerging here. Embrace that. And if you need to talk to someone, talk to someone. Reach out. Don't be alone if it's too painful. You have just started a brand new life. Let's do everything we can to make it the best one yet.

It's amazing how good those purees tasted. But it was also amazing to me how little I could usually palate. Only twice since starting on purees did I consume a full 1/2 cup of food. When I hadn't, it was usually somewhere around 3-5 table-spoons of food. Eating too much or too fast just felt like a bowling ball working its way down my throat. Oh, and that elephant would come back, too.

Now. Let's talk potatoes. I tried some. They tasted wonderful with a little pat of butter. However they may have been too starchy for me because about 90 minutes later I experienced my first ever bout of dumping syndrome.

You may have heard of it and think you know what it means, but you're wrong. Most people assume it's simply immediate diarrhea. It's not. In fact it doesn't even have to include diar-rhea as a symptom. It can. But not always. And not for me with those potatoes.

What happened was I had about three tablespoons of mashed potatoes and I was full. When the swelling did go down and my throat would settle, it would get easier and the quantities increased slightly. But for now, that three tablespoons was enough.

About 90 minutes later I was hit with a massive wave of nausea. It hit me like a freight train, fast and hard. A cold sweat washed over me and I started to get a little light headed. Within a minute I was soaked through with sweat, and I was starting to see double. I slowly moved to the couch and put my head back and tried not to vomit. It lasted about 30 minutes and then I was fine after some time and a protein shake. But it sucked, no doubt about it.

That had been the big thing I really had to learn through this. I was relearning how my body consumed food and liquid. I was taking sips and nibbles. But strangely, they seemed to be satisfying me so far. Which made no sense to me. Remember me? The guy who could put away a Hawks Box from McDonalds for dinner? But being satisfied with a few tablespoons of food in a sitting, in fact, was happening. So I just decided to roll with it.

CHAPTER 16

Being Supported - and Supportive

In the first two weeks post surgery, I lost 21.8 pounds. That's an amazing number in such a short time. My throat had become a little easier to get liquid down and I was able to tolerate a full 1/2 cup of food or one cup of liquid at a time. After two weeks on pureed food (think baby food), I moved on to "mechanical soft" food, which is mushy stuff you can cut with a fork. But something with substance. I kind of couldn't wait.

I want to discuss support with you. Being supported and having people to look to and rely on is key in any significant life altering change. Especially since there's a significant likelihood that you're not always going to feel wonderful about the change you're going through. I know I haven't.

See, about a week after the surgery I decided to weigh myself two days in a row. And I saw zero change on the scale. Zero. After eating less than 800 calories per day. And the surgery. Wasn't I supposed to be melting? Wasn't this surgery some amazing magic wand? I wasn't sleeping well, and insomnia is a ridiculous mistress that does crazy things to your perception of the world.

For example, while watching an episode of *Friends* on Nick at Nite (don't judge) I saw Joey eating a pastrami sandwich. While sipping my liquid and puree diet, I thought to myself "*I'll never get to ever eat a pastrami sandwich ever again.*" Which made me angry and sad. Combine that with the lack of weight loss and all of a sudden I felt like a failure again. I felt like the same failure that had failed at diet after diet and would never get thin and healthy and, on top of that, now had surgical scars to go with my failure as a scarlet letter emblazoned forever on my chest. Er...abdomen.

And in that dark place in my mind I turned to the Facebook support group that was established through Eviva for perspective. These people have been wonderfully supportive and helpful through this whole process. So find yourself a group. Find yourself some support. And if you can't find support or don't know who to talk to, I invite you to email me directly. I have no qualms with you calling out to me for support and caring no matter what your problem is. I'll try to listen and be there for you, as others have been there for me.

jonathan@sleevelifebook.com

To give you a glimpse into the type of support that I received in my doldrums, I informed my friends that I'd be sharing some of the comments here with you.

"Your body is working hard to figure out the changes. It will take time. You are doing extremely well!!"

"Stay the course you are doing great!"

"There will be times when you feel insecure and feel as though it takes an eternity, but then, one day, you will look at the numbers, and think, "Holy crap! It's happening!" Don't get discouraged!"

"How long did it take to get to 400 plus pounds? With that said it will take a little while for the weight to come off. Give yourself a break and work on healing."

"Do not beat yourself up. Your body has no choice but to lose weight."

"This weight loss is permanent. Every time you lose five pounds, you'll never see them again."

"Our disease (obesity) has conditioned us to think the worst (of course I would fail at weight loss surgery). Don't let yourself down. This works, just not on your timeline. The days and weeks you don't lose, your muscles are still getting stronger, your blood pressure is regulating, your life is being saved. When you do freak out, just reach out to us. We'll reel you back in."

So if you need to be reeled back in, reach out to the people around you and we'll reel you back in. And if you see someone you care for needing to be reeled in, throw them a lifeline and hang on tight. You are going to get through this and reinvent yourself step by step. Just like I am. And we'll do it together.

CHAPTER 17

Faith

Faith. We must have it. I'm not talking about spirituality or religion here—although those things can be of vital importance to people. No, I'm talking about faith in our own strength and power. Faith in our decision making progress. Faith in the people who have supported us and our decisions to change.

About three weeks after surgery, in the Facebook group, I saw that someone who had surgery the same day I did (hey Keith! Shoutout!) was doing fantastic and, in fact, appeared to be ahead of me in weight loss (I was at 22.6 pounds down in only 21 days). Because I am who I am, I decided to check my weight *again* that day and of course was the same as the day before, which I decided was a plateau. Two days is a plateau to me. I can be my own worst enemy.

Then my rational mind kicked in. Let's look at the facts here. According to the math everyone who has ever dieted knows from the Mayo Clinic (a clinic that makes Mayo? Awesome!) because 3,500 calories equals about one pound (0.45 kilogram) of fat, you need to burn 3,500 calories more than you take in to lose one pound. So, in general, if you cut 500 calories from your typical diet each day, you'd lose about one pound a week (500 calories x 7 days = 3,500 calories).

According to the internet (which is always right), in order to maintain my then current weight of 367.2 pounds, I'd have to be taking in at least 3000 calories per day, likely more.

Here are my caloric intake recordings from four days at that time. 848, 697, 705, 655. These represent an approximation of my new every day intake. An average of 726.25 calories per day. Some 2250 calories *less* than I'd have needed to maintain my weight.

So why was I not losing the average 4.5 pounds every week I should be if I was eating this little? Was it because the universe is against me? Was I just going to be inherently unhealthy forever?

Nope...we're not going to get into that downtalk again. Because faith, my friends.

Faith in science, math, and dedication. The numbers are sound. If you follow the plan you've set out for your change and it's a solid one, over time your reality will have no choice but to change to meet your goals. The key there is *over time*. One day, two days, three days, even a week—they're cosmic snapshots. Big picture you'll see the scale moving in the right direction, the changes you want to happen will happen, and you'll gain what you wanted out of life.

I could have been retaining water because soup has a lot of salt. I could have been constipated (forget could have been, I *was*) and retaining…well…poop. My metabolism could have still been at an all time low because of how sedentary recovery was (and it was time to get more active). My body could have just been screwy because we *took a piece out of it* and it was still adjusting.

Regardless, I stopped worrying. I gave up on panic and stress about it. Because I had faith. I believed that if I did the work, the results would come to me. My body would literally have no choice but to do what I wanted it to. I would continue the plan and have faith in the people I trusted, and most importantly, faith in myself.

I would have faith in something I hadn't had faith in for years. I would choose to believe in me.

I actually believed that I. WOULD. SUCCEED.

CHAPTER 18

Listen to Your Body

A lot changed for me in the first month after surgery and there was even more goodness waiting for me just around the river-bend (Thanks Pocahontas!).

Let's just recap the success at that point. The day I went in for my surgical consultation with Dr. Smooth Jazz himself I weighed 405 (gasp) pounds.

The day I had surgery I weighed 390 pounds.

One month after the surgery I weighed in at 354 pounds. I'd lost 51 pounds in about six weeks. And it felt amazing. Physically and emotionally I felt like I was really starting to come into my own.

But that didn't mean I wasn't still learning new things about #sleevelife. My sleeve was constantly teaching me things my brain didn't know anymore. See, for 38 years I've learned how to eat a meal and what a meal *looks* like.

My sleeve now formally disagreed with my brain.

So let's talk about retraining your mind and heart in the wake of any major life change and success. You have to not only make the change in terms of your actions, but also your thoughts. If your mind doesn't follow your body, nothing's going to stick. Let's give you a concrete example.

I took my adorable daughter out for breakfast one weekend. She ordered her normal french toast. I ordered two very soft scrambled eggs with a small sprinkling of cheddar cheese atop. That's it. Figured that was about what a serving would be for me at this point instead of the chicken fried steak and eggs with toast and hash browns I used to eat.

I ate half of it and was full. And full is a different feeling now. Full used to be pressure in my abdomen. Nope. Now it's pain in my sternum. And I don't mean a mild ache or dull throb. I mean sharp *"there's an elephant sitting on your sternum and pressing on your ribs"* pain. It's literally my body saying "DUDE—STOP—WE'RE FULL" in an extremely forceful way. It's not hard to listen if you know what the signal is. Usually that's followed by some hiccuping, which is just another signal in case I miss the first one.

So what signals are you receiving? Knots in your stomach? Pulse racing? Anxiety? Sure, maybe you didn't have weight loss surgery, but you're still retraining your body and brain to think and do things differently now.

Listen to yourself. Listen to your body and learn to understand the warnings and the pitfalls. You can succeed at this, just like me. We're doing it together, right? And learn to celebrate every single victory. Whether it's a pound lost or a mile walked or a job well done. Celebrate. You deserve it.

CHAPTER 19

How to Be Inspirational

I had my six week postoperative checkin with mental health and nutrition. They were now encouraging me to eat *more* calories than I had been. Which was going to be really really hard because I just got full so easily. About 900-1000 calories a day and I was stuffed. Which explained why, at six weeks postop, I was down over 68 pounds. Which felt amazing.

But at that checkup, something *truly* amazing happened. I received feedback on this very book. Rather, I received feedback on the idea behind this book. I was just standing at the counter buying some new protein laden snacks and someone approached me.

"Hi. You don't know me, but I'm following your posts on the Facebook group and I wanted to say thanks for posting parts of your book and just being there. You're a total inspiration!" And she introduced herself and I recognized her name and thanked her profusely for telling me. While doing that an Eviva employee approached me and called me by name, and I suddenly realized she was also a Facebook group member who posted frequently.

I explained to her that the woman had just introduced herself out of the blue and how awesome that felt. I always felt the need to use my personality and my ability to relay stories to people to help them relate and inspire. Hence my passion for this book you're holding in your hands (or your iPad or Kindle or whatever).

I'm not bragging. (#humblebrag?) No really. I'm not. I'm telling you how amazing it can feel to know your words or actions are helping others around you who may be struggling. It's a life changing experience and feeling, and once you feel it, you get greedy for it. You want it all the time. It changes who you are at your core. You go from just existing to thriving and wanting those around you to thrive.

So I challenge you, dear reader, to do it. Find someone to inspire. Even if it's your own family or even your pet. Find someone who looks at you and says "thank you" because if I can do it, you can do it. And so can they. Maybe the way out of the situation our world has found itself in isn't in our government's hands, but our own. Maybe if we just went out of our way to try and find things about ourselves that inspire our fellow citizens and encourage them to be their best, maybe it really would start to turn around.

Just food for thought.

Although this chapter is called "how" to be inspirational, not "why". So how do you do it? How can you find That Thing about yourself to inspire others? Well, maybe you just already know what it is, in which case, skip ahead to the next chapter.

The rest of you, I have a novel concept for you in order to find out the best things people in your life truly think about you.

Ask them.

Now stop complaining. It's not rude and you're not fishing for compliments. It's a legitimate way to get feedback on who you are and where your strengths lie. Ask your best friend, or your spouse, or your children, or whomever: "Is there something about me that inspires you?" I guarantee you there's a yes answer coming your way.

Once you know what it is, you can dial it up to eleven and use that inspirational power you *already* have to push others forward.

CHAPTER 20

Basics - Kids - Rewards

Basics. I want to discuss basics.

Success breeds success. But it also breeds complacency. It's easy once you start to succeed to rest on your laurels and believe you know what you're doing and to just start coasting. Which actually happened to me about two months after the surgery.

It was July 4, and I weighed in first thing in the morning to find out that I was down just shy of SEVENTY-FIVE pounds on this journey. I felt awesome and was confident in my abilities to keep this train rolling. I took myself out to breakfast. Then went out to lunch with a friend after a movie. I wasn't sure what the "content" of my lunch was so I didn't track it. Then I headed to a different friend's place for the traditional July 4th BBQ. Lots of smoked meats and lovely platters.

I didn't eat much, but I sure as heck ate more than I had in the last few weeks. Mainly because I spread dinner over two meals since there was food all day. Did I track any of it? Of course not.

Now some good news: I was far more physically able to do things than I had been in awhile. I played lots of bocce—the traditional July 4th competition game. I had a blast with all the families and kiddos that were there.

Now the bad news. I decided the next morning to weigh in and see what happened. Especially since I had no idea what I'd actually consumed.

I was up about a pound and a half.

But I wasn't disheartened. Nor should I have been. I knew going into the 4th that I was likely risking a small backslide. I hoped I wouldn't backslide, but then again, life has to be lived. So what would I do next?

This is where basics come into play. I went back to the basics of how and why I made the change in the first place. Let's consider that a second. If you try to make a change in life and start to succeed it's very important to keep track of it. You need to document it somehow because if you happen to backslide, you'll have no way to rein it back in and keep on track. It's easy to derail if you weren't keeping track of your path. Studies have, in fact, shown that people who track their progress towards a goal are much more likely to be successful.

Thankfully I had been tracking all along. So what did I do? I went back to five to six small meals throughout the day. I focused on protein. I tracked every bite. There's a great acronym I learned through all of this: ABC. All Bites Count. And I focused on keeping that pattern again going forward. I gave myself a week to see what sort of progress I could make with the change.

You can do it too. Refocus and succeed. Just like at the start, we'll do it together. Ready? Go!

While you're refocusing let's talk rewards, because why struggle if there aren't rewards? Oh yeah, and the most rewarding thing of for me...my kid. Let's talk about kids.

Kids. I have one. I love her. But some of them are pains in the neck, let's be honest.

The kid in question is one I met around two months post surgery at a community swimming pool. My kiddo and she had started playing together, and the girls decided I looked a lot like a jungle gym and started climbing on me.

The kid said "You're hairy." That's true. I'm Italian. It comes with the pasta.

Then she said "You're fat!" Her dad, who I'd been discussing my weight loss surgery with, immediately grabbed her and told her she couldn't say things like that. She didn't seem to understand.

"But he is!"

Now, two things surprised me in this interaction. First, my initial response was to say, out loud, "Not anymore!" Which is something I haven't *felt* in a very long time. Her dad explained to her that you can't just say things, even if they're true, and let's face it, I may have been down over 80 pounds, but I was still over 300 pounds total weight, so she wasn't really wrong. He also explained that I'd been working really hard and doing really well. She apologized, although I'm not sure she understood why.

But the second thing that surprised me was this. As the little girl had this conversation with her dad, my own daughter swam to me, sat on my knee, put her arms around my neck and kissed my cheek. She then whispered in my ear. "I think you look great, Daddo." (She calls me Daddo, because I call her Kiddo.) And I melted into the pool. Some kids don't know what to say. Some kids just do.

Okay, kids done. Let's talk rewards.

We gain the greatest rewards through personal journeys and evolving changes in our own world. Our own lives. In other words, the things that let us know we're actually succeeding. Oh wait. You thought I was going to start talking about food rewards and cheat days, didn't you? Hell no. That's how I got to where I was in the first place. Too much justification of the wrong food with "I deserve this."

When I started this journey I was 405 pounds. I was on three blood pressure medications, two anti-depressants, and a potassium supplement. Two months and change after surgery I went and saw my doctor because I'd been getting light headed when I stood up. Anyone who's ever had low blood pressure will tell you that this is a symptom of that condition.

Sure enough, my pressure had lowered to the point where we had to remove medications. Including an anti-depressant. I was then only on one blood pressure medication and one antidepressant. Which meant every morning when I went into the bathroom to get ready for the day I got a lovely reminder of the fact that I was succeeding. It was a reminder that wasn't tied to the scale or a number. Just less crap I have to put in my body.

Which I guess is a nice metaphor for the whole process here. I got to put less crap in because I was getting healthier overall.

CHAPTER 21

A Conversation with Myself

Negative talk can be a killer. I don't just mean people saying negative things to you. Oh no. I mean the worst kind. Negative *self* talk. Which I was engaging in one morning around ten weeks after the surgery. So instead of motivating you, I needed a little help motivating me. Or rather, I decided to talk to you, dear reader, about my issues and hoped that in doing so you'd help me through them by using you as my voice into myself so that you could see me and find yourself in me and we could do this together.

Or…something like that.

I'd been super happy because I was down 80 pounds and was off medication and everything. Except that I'd also been a little lax on things. Like on the 4th of July. A few family issues and a few BBQs and a few other excuses I'm sure I can come up with (that alien invasion really threw me for a loop). I hadn't been going hog wild in any sense and I hadn't eaten anything that I shouldn't. But I felt like I'd been eating more than I should a little. I mean, I was still topping out at like 1200-1400 calories a day, which should just have the weight melting off.

But the scale hadn't moved more than .2 pounds up or down in four days. So instead of remembering that my body was still adjusting to a major change less than three months ago, I just assumed that I'd done something wrong. And began looking for every single place I could have gone wrong.

I identified one and so it became my new "beat myself up" mantra. Exercise. I was cleared for weights and full exercise weeks prior. I walked sometimes. But not regularly. I'd cleaned out my exercise room at home and had an elliptical and a set of free weights. Had I used them? Of course not.

Some *Survivor* I was.

So instead I decided to use you. We've gotten to know each other a bit through this and I think I knew what you'd say to me.

Alright now, cut that crap out. Let's get down to brass tacks. You should be exercising and you know it. You want to. You even downloaded apps to do it.

But you're not used to doing it. You've been not exercising for longer than you can remember. No more using that as an excuse. Are you following your diet plan?

Are you tracking what you're doing?

Do you see the problem there? You're not being consistent. So first step, quit looking for excuses and just be consistent. Do what has worked.

Track everything that goes in. All Bites Count. Even at a restaurant or a BBQ...track it.

That'll alleviate any guilt you feel about "doing this wrong" - and for the record - you're down over 80 freaking pounds. How about a little pat on the back for yourself. You've worked super hard on this and are reaping the benefits. Life is hard. Anything worth doing is hard. Especially if it's a major life change - which you're going through.

As for exercise, it's just like the surgery decision. Just make a decision. Then take a logical step. Don't worry about a lifting regime or how much you'll be able to lift or how ripped your arms will be. Just make a decision. And start it.

Before you know it a month will have gone by. Then three months. And you'll be doing it without thinking. Kind of like portioning your food. You used to struggle and now it's almost second nature.

And when you get lazy, go back to basics. Seriously, do you even read the things you write? Then how about you borrow a little bit of the inspiration you're trying to send my way and use it for yourself.

Even when I feel like I'm failing, I'm always thinking about it. Changing the neural pathways and making new and better decisions. Learning how to live this new life of mine. Which is really what this is all about. Step by step learning. Celebrating every step, even if it's a half step backwards. Now it's up to us to take the next logical, giant step forward. Into our future.

CHAPTER 22

Giving Back

A lot of exciting things were happening for me as I approached 100 days out from surgery, and I want to use this moment to talk to you about them and how to capture them for yourself. We talked earlier about inspiration, how you can be inspiring to others and how you should.

But now let's talk about giving back. We don't exist in a vacuum. Often there are those worse off than us who need our help. I think back to my father's words: "*I envied a man who had shoes when I had none. Until I saw a man who had no feet.*" I think you get the point. So how do we use our personal growth stories and motivation to catapult us into helping others?

Star Wars, of course. Specifically the Dark Side.

Okay, that's how I'd decided to do it, but you don't have to. Here's what I'm talking about.

One of my fitness goals had always been to get back into RunDisney Half Marathons. And in April 2017, RunDisney was doing a Star Wars Dark Side challenge at Walt Disney World.

This included a ten kilometer race on Saturday followed by a half marathon on Sunday.

And I registered and was going to do it. Because *Star Wars* and Disney. Also health.

But how was that about giving back?

Well, years ago when I lost a bunch of weight and started half marathoning, I raised a bunch of money through that process for Make-a-Wish, remember? And it was time to use that motivation to push forward. I'd decided to start raising charity dollars again. I wasn't sure how I'd be doing it or for which charity (either Make-a-Wish or Give Kids the World), but the idea was already percolating in my head and starting to generate positivity, which breeds positivity.

So, how are you going to use the newfound energy and life force you've found through your change to help others? What can you do for them? How are you going to challenge yourself to be better today than you were yesterday and how can you give that to others?

It doesn't have to be charity at all! It can just be positivity. I'm thinking of a young lady in our Facebook group who posts videos of incredibly inspiring messages for all of us on a nearly daily basis. And she's reaping the rewards because she's getting the feedback from us that it's helping. So she succeeds more and we succeed more and it builds like a feedback loop.

And she's not even using *Star Wars*. So surely you can do something too.

Do it. I challenge you.

CHAPTER 23

Small Victories

I'd just returned from a trip to Hawaii. This was a monumental trip for me. And it was time to start celebrating my successes. And yours. Recognizing your worth. Cheering yourself on.

Let's see what I had to celebrate, because you know it's not just the big stuff. Sometimes it's little stuff.

For instance, this was the first trip I'd taken in years where I didn't need to request a seat belt extension on my flight.

I was able to eat food prepared by the restaurants at the resort and actually lose weight because my mind was retrained on how to eat and what a portion is for me.

Just before leaving I had to buy five new suits because of the weight I'm losing so rapidly. They fit very nicely.

Oh yeah, and I was down 97.6 pounds so far. In just shy of 100 days since surgery.

I walked around Hawaii not embarrassed to be in a swimsuit. I tried out a water slide that I'd done before. Last time I'd had to occasionally help myself along. This time I shot through it like a bullet and nearly tore my own head off when I hit the water. It was a very different experience to say the least.

Now, I was nowhere near done with this journey. Nor am I anywhere done with this book. We're going through to one full year post surgery.

There were of course downs to counterbalance the ups, too. I was starting to wonder about the negative impact of sagging skin post surgery. I wasn't sure if I liked what I was seeing in the mirror.

But now I had a more positive mindset than ever before and so I just resolved to work on it by exercising more. Seeing what I could accomplish.

Success breeds success. The more you accomplish on your journey, the more your mindset changes and adapts to the "new you."

I'd started believing in the possibility that this may be an actual lifelong change—that I might just actually succeed at this. Because I already was. So celebrate your successes. Find something you've done right and shout it from the rooftops today. If you can't find something, then celebrate that you're *looking* for something to celebrate. Every step counts. Every moment works. Every second is a chance to inspire yourself to live a better second after that.

That's what this is all about. Betterment. For you and yours.

CHAPTER 24

Dating, Libido, and Sleeving

Being single is something we've all been through from time to time. Maybe it's all we ever know. When I made my decision to have surgery, I was single. As I'm writing this, I still am. But I've done some dating along the way. It's been interesting and hard and scary and fun and amazing.

I'm sure you're thinking that a big part of why it's been so interesting is all the weight I've lost. Yes, that's a part, but it's not the entirety of it all. In fact, it's not even a big part.

The thing is, as you go through a major life shift and begin to reevaluate yourself, you experience a variety of changes, not just the ones you had originally thought or intended. You consider your past, your present, and your future. What I've come to realize is that although I crave and desire a partner and mate, I'm not yet a version of me that can truly be an equal partner. I'm still evolving every day.

Although I was already divorced when I chose to have the surgery, did you know that post weight loss surgery divorce rates are 80-85% in the first two years after the surgery? According to the research it has to do with increased self-esteem, higher confidence, feelings of accomplishment, and enhanced energy.

The reality is that I find myself confident in ways I never was before. This confidence turns into taking much larger risks when dating and/or meeting people. Talking to women when I wouldn't have had the courage to even approach them before. Now let me be very clear: I am not a shallow individual. I'm not specifically referring to people who are traditionally more or less attractive. I simply mean that before my surgery I wouldn't even approach a woman in person. I'd assume they'd just have no interest. Because I saw myself as unwanted and unloveable. Undeserving.

Which is a load of crap. I wasn't. I was a great guy. But I didn't see it or believe it. Couldn't see it or believe it. I was mired in the muck of self doubt, and couldn't do anything to get out of it.

All of a sudden, every day I was seeing and feeling a different, better, happier, healthier me. It showed in every selfie I took and every new piece of clothing I tried on. It didn't hurt that friends and co-workers (and in some cases strangers) were telling me how much of a change they see in me. The thing they were always commenting on—especially if they'd known me awhile—wasn't the weight loss, but rather the smile. The confidence.

So what do you do with your newfound confidence? That smile? Well the first thing you do is immediately try to find someone to share it with. Maybe even like minded folks who've been through a similar transformation.

Let me caution you. This could be a major mistake. It was for me. You see, I wasn't ready. I still had to deal with the emotional baggage and pain from my past that had gotten me into the mess that led to this journey. So I inadvertently hurt a lot of people. They'd grow attached to me, and because I wasn't ready, I'd shun that attachment and they'd end up getting hurt. I'd like to take a moment to say publicly that I'm sorry for this. At the time, I honestly didn't realize how not ready I was.

After what I've experienced, I'd advise you really look hard at yourself. Are you in a situation where you are able to (and want to) take on a relationship at this point in your life? You're spending so much time focusing on getting through this change for you, creating the best you possible, and that takes up a lot of your energy. So don't rush. Get to a point where you really have what's needed to commit to something big like a relationship. Dating casually, however, if that's your thing… totally different story. Enjoy that, but be honest and straightforward with people. You have an obligation to consider others in your journey. At first you might think it's all roses and unicorns, but it can hurt those who get caught in your wake. So if you're honest and straightforward and let them make their own decisions, great. But go slow. And above all, follow your heart. You will know when you're ready. And until then, just be real with others and yourself. Be careful and be caring. Most of all to you.

Another cautionary tale. This one may be unique to weight loss surgery, but I'm not entirely sure of that. I've done an informal survey of friends who have undergone weight loss surgery and many of us are dealing with it. It deals with libido.

Since the surgery, our sex drives have been through the roof. Massively out of control. So much so that it's easily one of the first topics of conversation in many circles.

This tale will be short and sweet, because I don't kiss and tell and this is not Amy Schumer's book (which by the way was amazing...love you, Amy! Let's do lunch!). Be careful. With yourself. With your heart. With the hearts of others. You may think you can have casual sex, and you may even be right, but unless you're being very very straightforward about your intentions, you run a lot of risks. I'm not saying it can't work. It can be fun, if both parties are clear on where they stand. But you have to be honest and careful.

Let's look at some of the risks:

- Emotional damage
- Unwanted attachments (for you or for them)
- Complicated relationships
- STIs
- Unwanted pregnancy
- Crazy people stalking you on Facebook and messaging your friends to tell them awful things about you... or maybe that one was just me.

So go have fun and, as always, follow your heart. Not your groin. Or *do* follow your groin, but listen to your conscience along the way. And remember that honesty thing.

It's been brought to my attention that this section of the book is decidedly depressing, despite sexuality being just a wonderful part of the human experience. And an even more won-derful part of the experience after losing over 160 pounds. So despite my earlier proclamation that I wouldn't be kissing and telling, I'm going to relate to you a single story about my own sexual history in the wake of this surgery. One that will explain just what a change my world, body, and libido have been through.

I should preface this by telling you that I've struggled with some severe anxiety surrounding sexuality and attachment and relationships. So this was a pretty big decision for me at this point. I actually hadn't had intercourse since prior to the surgery (and in fact, due to my size, wasn't successful in over a year), and this was now six months post surgery. I'll come back to the anxieties and fears later in this book. Don't get upset. Yes, the libido conversation was still accurate and about me, but being sexual and having intercourse are not necessarily the same thing to everyone.

I had been dating a woman for a bit and we'd decided to go ahead and have sex. When we got to the moment, I stopped cold. And for the first time in my life I was able to actually see what was happening between me and a woman. My stomach wasn't in the way and I could see and feel and so much more. The fat pad around my groin had shrunk as well, so I felt stronger and more virile, and I could see it all.

What an amazing feeling.

CHAPTER 25

Stalls

It happens to the best of us. We set goals. We work hard. We succeed. And then, despite our best efforts, the success just stalls. Stagnates. We stop. We plateau. And then we all do pretty much the same thing.

We obsess.

We criticize ourselves.

We wonder what we did wrong.

And then, if we've ever struggled with these issues before, we end up sitting in a dark room with a pint of high protein ice cream and a stomach ache telling ourselves it'll all get better in the morning. Then we lay in bed and wonder if the fact that we had a bad night will undo every single bit of hard work we've done and that we'll just wake up and be fat again overnight magically.

The reality is that any change takes time. All races are marathons, not sprints. I know that some races are *in fact* sprints, but even those are marathons. They're just fast ones.

Every race, every goal, every change and project is a matter of stepping forward towards a finish line. Sometimes we stumble and fall. What matters is that we get back up and keep moving forward.

Let me give you an example.

One-hundred-thirty pounds gone was a major milestone for me. Not that there's anything special about that number, but at 275 pounds, I was officially smaller than I'd ever been in my adult life. That felt amazing. I actually had people who knew me professionally and didn't recognize me. But then...I held there—stopped—stuck around 273-275 and fluctuating back and forth for a few weeks. In fact, as I'm writing at this moment I'm still there. Stuck. (Spoiler Alert Author's note: I made it through!)

And yes, I've had moments of weakness where I've overeaten or eaten an extra meal late at night. Things that I did solely because they just made me feel a little bit better about myself and my struggle. And then I instantly felt badly about them. Not just emotionally mind you. I felt badly physically too, because remember there's less real estate inside me.

So how did I cope with it? I remembered the past—the struggles—and compared them. A pint of high protein ice cream is about 280 calories. A McDonalds Hawks Box, (called a Blitz Box in other areas, but since I'm from the Pacific Northwest it's all about the Seahawks! GO HAWKS!) which was my "I'm pissed off" snack of choice pre-surgery, has over 2900 calories. Over TEN TIMES as many. And I could down one with no problem and chase it with a pint of Ben and Jerry's. Now I struggled to even get to the bottom of the low calorie protein laden ice cream.

So okay, first step to getting through a stall - is to just recognize that if you're reverting to coping mechanisms - that you're at least trying to cope in a more healthy way.

What else? You look for other changes you can make. Me? I had a bike now. And an elliptical machine. And was training for a 10k/half marathon challenge. And was auditioning for Survivor. Yeah, I had all those things, but when I hit this stall, I finally decided to actually *use* them. And I knew that my body was preparing to blast through this stall. I just had to keep doing what I was doing and working hard. It's how I got as far as I was at that point.

The reality is that it didn't take me only six months to get fat. It sure as hell was going to take me more than six months to get skinny and healthy. And there was going to be stalls and peaks and valleys and ups and downs and lefts and rights and every other metaphor you can think of. So how do you maintain a change?

By recognizing that the real change is inside your mind. It's about finally believing you can achieve your dreams and your goals, trusting in that belief and working hard to make sure that belief manifests into reality.

CHAPTER 26

Enjoying Sunshine

By the time I'd made the decision to have surgery, I was truly mired in a depression. If you've never felt or been clinically depressed let me share with you a little of how it feels and what it's like.

My world was a place where nothing felt doable other than what I was already familiar with. I could watch TV. I could work. I could even play video games. Oh yeah...and I could eat. That I could really do. And it was comforting. No matter how much I couldn't control what my body felt or how much my back hurt or the cramps in my side when I moved, I could control what went into my mouth.

You'd think that would make it easy to make a change and put *less* in. Quite the opposite. Nobody was going to tell me what I could and couldn't eat. It was the one area where I was allowed to do things solely because they felt good.

I was always warm and sweating. I kept my air conditioner cranked to 58 degrees in my house just to be comfortable. I kept the blinds drawn and the lights off. My daughter frequently referred to my home as my "cave". She saw me like a bear and my heart was truly hibernating. My relationships suffered. When I did try to date, it would be quick and relatively arms length for me (and yes, if you dated me during this time, I'm sorry). Dating someone left me feeling even more alone.

But the food was always there. Always. And the cave. My cave.

I was keeping a daily journal of my "exercise" and "mood". This was at the urging of my primary care doctor and counselor. They suggested that this would help me keep track of everything I was doing and how I was feeling about it. I keep this journal and recently went back and re-read parts of it. I'm reprinting parts of it here so that you can see exactly where I was physically and emotionally before all this went down.

"Walked to concert with Amber. Sat together. Long walk up hills and stairs. Hurt my back. And my lungs. Ugh."

"Did six minutes on my elliptical before picking up kiddo. Had the time, figured I'd do it. Back and butt and hamstrings hurt."

"Doing zero minutes this morning because I just don't want to. I know I'll be walking a lot downtown later today and I'm rationalizing it that way. If I recognize that, shouldn't I be able to just get off my ass and exercise? Except I don't want to right now."

"Did seven minutes. Side stitch and sweating."

"Mild moment of chest pain. Like a small muscle cramp. What I used to think of as my heart skipping a beat. Happened

when I was a kid. Mentioned it to dad. No worries. Still happens sometimes. Worried about my health and so I'm fretting a little. Plus the things on me that never quite heal, but I do pick. Bad circulation? Or do I have some rare cancers growing all over me? Unlikely. But what if. I'm not ready to even think about death. Death scares me. A lot. Wednesday night at the movies, guys sat right behind me and I actually spent moments wondering if they were killers and trying to figure out if they shot me right through the back of my head what I'd feel and where I'd go. It was scary. So I stopped. I'm somewhat able to stop when things like that happen. Maybe I should mention the chest pain to Dr. Zeh. Or would I end up at a cardiologist? Should I be? Gah. I'm getting all wrapped up in anxiety again. Then fretting about little stuff. Like when should I buy new clothes? I have zero long sleeve sweaters or casual wear that fits because I'm too fat which is why my chest hurts and why I shouldn't shop because I'm just not worth it."

"I feel bloated. Tired. Run down. My body hurts to move. I get winded going up a flight of stairs. I'm a mess. I really do need to rebuild myself."

"Heart beating in my throat. Continued throughout dinner. Looked up palpitations and angina and whatnot online. Seems consistent with the occasional chest pangs I get. And it's likely nothing at all. Like 99%. But also could be super serious. Slightly more convinced than ever that I'll collapse and die in Disney all alone and no one will know. Fighting that generalized anxiety. Which is hard when you can feel your heart beating in your throat."

"I shouldn't be out of breath walking a hallway with a grocery bag. I should and want to be better than this."

"I'm surrounded by racers. All talking about the races and how they felt and did and running and medals. And I haven't even said congratulations to anyone I see yet. I just feel like I'd owe an explanation of how and why a big fat guy knows about marathon medals. *sigh* There's that negativity again. Grrrrrr."

"I couldn't help feeling like the fat guy. I had trouble sitting in the tight seats at the theatre and being comfortable. When I was on stage I felt like my ass was on display and was huge because somehow I ended up with my back to the audience every time. And squatting. Just more motivation to change."

"Tuesday 2/16/16. Called what used to be Puget Sound Bariatrics to get information. I'm a little nervous about seeing my doctor today. Not sure why. But just am. I can feel my anxiety level rising already. Pressure was decent here. But weight clocked in at 405 pounds. Holy hell. I don't even know how to process that number. Or what it even means. No wonder my back hurts and I'm sweaty all the time. What are we going to do about this? Doc says it's time to really consider the surgery. I'm hard pressed to disagree. It's time. I'm gathering information and we'll meet again in 3-4 weeks to discuss. She says I'm going about this the right way and doing so methodically. And that dad would be proud. Which of course got me all misty."

It amazes me just how much difficulty I was having moving around and how awful my emotional state really was. I was struggling so much even seeing myself as worth making a change. Until that appointment on February 16th, when I made the decision that altered the course of my life forever.

After my surgery my mood started to change. Not just because of the physical changes I was going through, but because I was starting to see value in myself again. I was starting to see myself as someone who could be loved and cherished by me. I was becoming the best version of myself I'd ever been.

One day, about three months after my surgery, I realized a few things that were amazing to me.

First, I was sitting in my playroom watching TV. And I was chilly. Cold, in fact. I grabbed a blanket. When I went downstairs to get some iced tea I raised the temperature in the house. Now I still like it colder than some, but I keep it a nice comfortable 68. Up ten degrees. And I have blankets for when you come over to visit. (Which reminds me...when *are* you coming over? We've been through so much already I feel like it's time. Sheesh.)

Second, it was too dark. I opened the shades. Sunlight streamed into the room and across my face. I liked it. It took a little getting used to, but I liked it. I started enjoying going outside with my daughter. Going for walks. My back didn't hurt. My shins and calves didn't hurt. I could walk distances and enjoy it. I started getting to know some of my neighbors. I started coming out of my cave. Don't get me wrong, dark and night and gray and rain are still my favorites. They were long before the depression. I'm a night owl. My home office has blackout curtains because I work best in the dark.

But now I'm a bear who likes to go enjoy the daytime, too. When I stay in the dark it's not because I fear the light, it's because I like the dark.

And that brings me to fear. Which of course is the path to the dark side. Oops—my geek is showing again.

Fear of change is one of the most powerful fears there is. We know *now*. We are safe *now,* even if now sucks. Now is familiar. What's coming? That's scary because it could be damn near anything.

But as my depression lifts, the future seems less scary and more hopeful. It could be damn near anything!

It's amazing what happens when your chief coping mechanism disappears. You are forced to actually think your way through things and figure out why and how you're really feeling. If I couldn't eat my feelings, I was just going to have to feel them. Which believe it or not is the only way through them. You can't avoid your feelings. You have to go *through* not around. The journey is just as valuable as the destination on this one…trust me.

Let me be clear. I didn't just bust through my depression without help. I was on anti-depressants and in weekly counseling (still am…hi Dayna!). These tools are what helped me develop the skills I needed to start to make my cave a little bigger and brighter. Cleaner. More open. More inviting.

It's still my cave and likely always will be. But it's just where I end up after having a great day. And even if I don't *go* anywhere that day, I'm still doing better than I was because sunshine is a good thing. Daylight is a good thing. Hope is a good thing.

Hope. And light.

CHAPTER 27

Baking and Bites

"Daddo! Let's bake!"

It was August 26th, 2016. One-hundred-fourteen days had passed since my surgery. That day was massively significant because it was the day I passed under 300 pounds and finally weighed just 299. I was down 106 pounds total and feeling like a million dollars. It was a huge success that morning.

And now she wanted to bake. *Oh dear Lord give me strength!* How was I supposed to do this? How could I support my little girl and be active with her in the kitchen and also support my own weight loss goals? I'd avoided anything even remotely resembling a sweet and now she wanted to friggin' *bake?!?*

Okay, maybe it's wasn't that dramatic. Let's get some information.

"Um. Sure kiddo. What should we bake?"

"Zucchini bread!" Not bad.

"Brownies and a cake too!" Oh crap.

The fundamental rule of improvisation is accepting the reality put to you with a hearty "yes, and". As an improviser, I knew there was only one way through this dilemma.

"You got it, Kiddo! Let's go walk around the store and pick what we need!" Maybe walking the store would help me buy time to figure a way out of this mess.

Sure enough two hours later we were back at the house with arms full of baking supplies. Cake mixes. Brownie mix. Fresh zucchini. A five pound bag of sugar. My inner fat guy was hyperventilating. So I turned where I had so many times for inspiration through this process. My Facebook group.

They encouraged me to simply try things. See how they tasted. See what my body did. They reminded me that this change wasn't some extreme diet or some journey that eventually ends and goes back to "normal." Nope. This was permanent. Part of my anatomy was *gone* and never coming back. Was I expecting to never eat cake for the rest of my days? I might as well see what happened today.

So we baked. I didn't lick or taste anything while we did. Kiddo got to lick every spatula. I was determined that if I was going to try things I'd measure them and try them when they were finished.

Which is precisely what I did.

I had a half ounce of zucchini bread. It was dense and thick and not at all what I expected it to be. But it was a nice change.

I cut a small, one inch squared corner of cake with a little dollop of frosting on it. That frosting was so sweet it made me pucker my lips and close my eyes, but the cake was moist and lovely.

I noticed something though. I was already filling up. I could feel the now familiar pressure in my upper chest that told me my stomach was just about done with things. But brownies! They're my favorite! And they were Ghirardelli! I had just enough room for a bite. But I'd want more. I'd likely cut too big a bite. And then I'd get fat again because I ate too big of a brownie bite one day. I'd undo the entire surgery just from this brownie bite. Which was a clue that my negative self talk was back rearing its ugly head.

How was I going to manage this? I knew what I wanted, but my fears were taking over, and my body couldn't really accommodate much more. I tried to focus my willpower into a solution as I cut the pan so they could cool and kiddo could have one.

As I pulled the butter knife from the pan of brownies a glob of ooey-gooey brownie came off with it. Stuck to the knife. About the size of a large grape. At the same exact moment both the angel and devil on my shoulders exclaimed "YES!" in unison. This was my answer.

I slowly and tentatively licked the glob and then bit into it. I took a moment and allowed the chocolatey goodness to just live on my tongue. When I swallowed it I realized that I was now full. I hadn't over eaten. And I'd tried every damn thing I'd baked.

I'd done it. I'd successfully done something I wondered how I was going to do for the last hundred days.

I'd *lived my life*. And I'd done so with my sleeve instead of in spite of it.

Which is really what I want you to do. Don't think of whatever change you're going through as something to overcome or conquer. Think of it as a new family member you just have to find a way to coexist and develop a healthy, strong relation-ship with...and occasionally share a brownie bite Something you can be proud of that helps you grow.

CHAPTER 28

Dehydration and Constipation

I'd decided that it was time to put my distance walking to the test. My office was exactly two miles from my home, and I knew a round trip would be four miles. Not a bad test of distance. I grabbed my headset and my iPhone playlist and headed out the door with excitement. I wanted to know how far I could go, and moreover, how fast I could get there.

Now, a side note is important here. This may surprise you to learn, but what goes into your body will *eventually* come out. Yes folks, I'm talking about poop. When you're taking in so few calories and most of them are protein based and very little fiber or roughage (there's no room), well, you just can't poop sometimes.

Not even the squatty potty helped.

I was just bound up. Badly.

So my nutritionist suggested that I do a few things. First we tried adding in some dried fruits (prunes specifically) every day. Not much, but some. Secondly I started adding MiraLax to my iced tea. A standard dose every bottle.

It helped a little bit over time. But movement will make things…well….move more.

Flash forward. I walked to my office and had a great time. It was a good, fun walk. I sat at my desk feeling accomplished and met with a client or two. And then it was time to walk home. I was excited about it, but the sun was higher in the sky and it was warmer. I was hot. And starting to sweat.

And I'd forgotten a water bottle.

About half way, I started to feel slightly lightheaded.

Shortly thereafter, my stomach started cramping mightily. My laxative was hitting me. All at once. I'd walked things through my system to the point that my system was ready to let go. Add the lightheadedness and I knew I was having trouble.

Between my house and my office there was nowhere to stop. I had to keep going. There was no option. I had to power through.

I flashed back to that half marathon in the Florida heat, when I had a massive bout of dehydration—those moments where I thought I was dying. My head was starting to feel like that. I was getting scared. My stomach was adding its loud crampy voice to the mix.

I actually worried that I would be subject to an accident and mess myself. But I kept walking. Powering. I had to get home. When I finally did, I grabbed for an Isopure protein water and ran to the bathroom. My body literally exploded at that moment.

Here's what I learned: preparation is important. A water bottle was a necessary tool for me now. I used to only need water on walks longer than seven miles. Now I'd need it early on. And I'd have to sip as I went.

But preparation really is the key. You'll have to learn how changes will affect you and the way you move forward in life. Learn the hard way if you like, but you might want to carry a change of boxers in the meantime.

CHAPTER 29

Not Being Recognized

"Good morning, Judge!"

I was in one of my favorite courtrooms about three months post-op and it was before the calendar had started for the day. The judge was on the bench. I'd known him for years and in fact spent three days a week with him in court when I was a public defender. For two years solid. He glanced up at me and mumbled something. He was busy. It happens.

I left the courtroom and chatted with my client for a few minutes. After that I came back in. The clerk immediately singled me out.

"Mr. Dichter? The judge would like to see you in chambers a moment."

This was unusual for me. Not unheard of, but unusual. Was I in trouble? I couldn't really tell what was going on. But I cheerfully stepped behind the bench and into the judge's office. He was smiling at me and extended his hand to shake mine.

"I owe you an apology."

He did?

"I'm sure you don't, Judge. But what for?"

"You shaved your head. And you lost weight. And you look totally different. You said hello and I looked up and at first glance I thought you were John Smith!" (*NOTE*: John Smith is *not* what the judge actually said. This judge had recently run for reelection as an incumbent candidate, which is a position almost nobody runs against, and his opponent was the attorney I'm renaming "John Smith" for these purposes.) Sufficed to say, he thought I was the guy who'd just run against him! Obviously the judge had won the election, but still, you don't run against a sitting judge!

"You just ran against me and now you're gonna come in here and say 'good morning, Judge' like nothing ever happened. Well, I told my clerk to find you another courtroom because I sure wasn't going to hear your case. She said 'Why? It's Dichter!' Well, I had absolutely no idea. I got a good laugh out of that. Have you ever considered wearing a nametag into my courtroom?"

You know, I hadn't considered it. Until that moment. It was also the first time someone who actually knows me had looked right past me and not seen the me they expected to see. It wouldn't be the last.

About six months post-op I had a client set for a jury trial. I hadn't seen her since just before the surgery. She and her mother walked *right past* me in the hallway. They were shocked when they realized.

I take frequent pictures of myself now. And by frequent I mean every single minute of every single day. You'd think I was a Kardashian the way I selfie myself. But it's different now. I like...no, I *love* the way I look. For the first time in...ever.

I've donated thousands of dollars of clothing and suits this year to various charitable organizations because about every three months I have to buy some new suits. They're wonderful. Let's consider that when I started this journey I was wearing jeans at a size 60. My jacket size was a 60-62 Long. My neck size was 22 inches.

Recently, I purchased some new suits. 48 Regular. New jeans. 40 inch waist. New dress shirts at 18 inches. Slim fit cut. What the heck is THAT? Slim fit? Me? The smallest professional clothing I'd ever owned.

Now, let's take a moment and discuss some pro tips on clothing shopping...or frankly doing anything to take advantage of incremental changes in yourself as you go on your journey.

NUMBER ONE: GO SLOWLY.

NUMBER TWO: See Number One.

See the thing is that the changes are just that...incremental. Which means that what fits perfectly today will be a little baggy tomorrow. What's tight today will be perfect tomorrow. What's already baggy will fall off your body leaving your underwear showing in the middle of a crowded store at the mall. Or something like that.

So take your time. Buy what you need only. And when you do, buy it for tomorrow, not yesterday. In other words ask them to tailor your suits a little snugger than you like. Because they are going to fit you perfectly within a short period of time.

You are changing. All of you. From top to bottom and inside and out. Enjoy the ride. Selfie the hell out of yourself. Invent new hashtags! Enjoy your rebirth and then find me and tell me how amazing you feel all over. Because sometimes I need to hear about *your* success to help me stay on *my* path.

CHAPTER 30

Testicular Terror

My doctor mentioned to me that it'd been about two years since we did a full physical. I was over six months post surgery and we decided that we'd go ahead and schedule a routine physical. I was excited. I'd felt better over the previous months than I had in years. I knew my pressure was down and normal. My blood work was showing normal. I was waiting for an amazing report.

We sat there and went through the entire physical and I was getting the stellar report I had been expecting. The last thing we were going to do was a testicular exam, because it's suggested at my age. No worries. Happy to do it.

"Hmmm. Have you had a vasectomy?"

Have I what? "No."

"Okay."

She was taking a little longer than I expected her to.

"Has this always been here? Do you check at home?"

Wait—what?

"Here. Feel here at the top of this testicle."

She moved my fingers to the area where I felt a small squishy pea sized lump. I actually felt my heart and stomach fall. *Oh shit.* I didn't know if it was or wasn't new.

"What is it?"

"I don't think it's anything. It's squishy, and usually if it's a problem it's hard as a rock. I'd say let's just watch and see if it changes. Check yourself at home from time to time."

"But what could it be, Doc?"

"Could be a variety of things. Could be a varicose vein, but I don't think so. Maybe just a backup of semen that'll clear on it's own. I doubt it's a tumor. I'm not worried."

Fuck. She said tumor. Words started floating through my mind. Cancer. Tumor. Surgery. Chemotherapy. I could feel my hand starting to shake.

"So really, we're not worried?"

"If I was worried, or if you're going to lose sleep over it, I'd send you for an ultrasound to show you there's nothing there."

Why didn't she just say, "Nope. Not worried. Don't be silly." That would have put me totally at ease. Mostly. Somewhat. Not really. But as it was, now I was starting to panic.

I asked her to refer me for an ultrasound. She said it would be at the lab in an hour. I called the lab two hours later. There was no referral yet. I called the doctor's office. They said they'd leave a message and get back to me. *Damn.* I just wanted this test done so I'd have peace of mind.

I put a post on Facebook in the group for my sleeve friends. Many suggested that it could just be a fatty deposit or cyst. As my body changed, things were revealing themselves. Everyone had been very supportive of the idea of getting the scan done.

The next morning I called the lab. Still no referral. So I stressed out and called my doctor again to get the referral sent. After several more hours, I got a call from the lab. My daughter was in the car and my speakerphone was on.

"We'd like to schedule your testicular ultrasound."

Talk about turning red. Thankfully my seven-year-old had no idea what the heck they were talking about. I wanted this thing done as quickly as possible. So I told her I had to have a medical test done and she'd have to come along with me. She smiled and agreed, having absolutely no idea what was happening, instead enthralled with her iPod.

I arrived for the ultrasound about 45 minutes later and was escorted into a room with a young female ultrasound technician. *Oh great. She's going to see my junk. Oh crap. She's going to feel my junk! Maybe we should chit chat? Get to know each other? Can I buy you a cup of coffee?*

"Go ahead and put this robe on. Do you want cool gel or warmed gel? Most people choose warmed, but it's different for everyone."

Wait. What? I had choices on the temperature of the goop a young female stranger is going to squirt on my scrotum in order to determine if I have testicular cancer? How was this even a thing? I wasn't sure how to respond so I nodded and weakly said, "warm". She stepped out of the room and told me to take off my pants and boxers and get on the table under the sheet.

Yep. Just like a massage table. That's what I kept telling myself. Except a massage of my scrotum. With a weird wand. And warmed goop. In the hands of a stranger.

As she manipulated my skin and flesh I stared at her face looking for any signs of recognition. I knew she was a technician and not the radiologist, but I also knew she knew what she was looking at. If I saw a flash of surprise or sadness I'd know. But she was hard to read.

"Okay, so I'm having a hard time seeing what she's concerned about. Do you know where it is? Or can you show me so I can feel it?"

Was she kidding me? Instead of her manipulating my junk, she wanted me to manipulate it for her and show her what my doctor had freaked me out about the day before? I sighed and attempted to find "it". When I did I pointed it out to her.

"Oh. That. That's small. Let me try to get a picture."

She looked nonplussed. As if this was truly no big deal. I felt my demeanor start to improve. When the pictures were taken, I spoke up.

"So? Tell me."

"I'm not a radiologist, Sir."

"I know. But tell me."

"Okay. I didn't see or feel anything that is concerning at all."

I breathed a massive sigh of relief. Sure enough a few days later the radiology report confirmed that I had a clogged gland that would work its way through and it was nothing to worry about. This was nearly a year post op, and the only medical complication I'd had since my abdominal surgery was a clogged gland in my junk. Now, two years post-op, I've had a couple of additional surgeries. As a result of the weight loss, my gallbladder developed two very large gallstones. It ended up coming out. Most recently, as a result of some hanging skin that I was unhappy with, I had a tummy tuck. Why document these adventures? Because they're part of the story, and they're part of the changes I've been through. And because they're part of who I am.

CHAPTER 31

Flying

All my life I've been a fan of super heroes. Comic books, movies, television shows, you name it. *Spider-man* has always been a favorite. But *Superman* holds a special place in my heart. Not only does he fight for truth, justice, and the American way, he possesses the ultimate set of powers: invulnerability, ice-breath, heat-vision, super-hearing, super-strength, kisses that erase memories and the ability to turn back time by spinning the planet backwards (yeah, thanks for *that* Mario Puzo...stick to gangsters), and of course, the ability to fly.

From the time I could walk, I was trying to fly. As a kid, we had a sunken living room—three steps down. We had a CD Player nearby and I'd play the theme from *Superman: the Movie* (because John Williams) as loud as it would go, and run and jump off those stairs, willing myself to fly into the air.

Of course it never happened. But in my mind it did a thousand times. In my dreams too. Flying dreams are one of my most common dreams. I adore the idea of being weightless and floating through the air on my own power. Zooming from place to place like a bird on the wind. John Williams music would be blaring behind me, of course. But it was a dream I never believed I'd truly achieve, especially as I grew both in terms of age and size.

As I approached eight months post surgery and my weight was around 265 pounds (the lowest weight I could remember at that time), I decided it was time to make this dream come true. Nearby Seattle is a very exciting venture that allows for indoor skydiving. I had no idea what it truly entailed, but I'd seen it from the highway and decided to check out the website.

Floating in a wind tunnel? Spinning and flipping and doing tricks? It's flying! It's really flying. And I was under the weight limit! I was going to do this! I wanted to fly for an hour or so! Maybe more!

"Okay, so our suggested beginning package includes four minutes of flight time."

Four minutes!? No no. I want hours!

"It'll be broken into four, one-minute segments in the tunnel."

One minute at a time! Are you kidding me?

"Trust me, Sir, one minute is a long time in the tunnel, especially for someone who's a first timer."

Committed to my four minutes of dreamtime, I signed myself and my daughter up to go indoor skydiving. She was very excited for the adventure with her dad, and as we headed to the facility I felt myself getting excited for what awaited me. We got there, purchased the suggested upgrades (enclosed helmet, a "high fly", and some photos) and watched a group before us.

Rather than describe to you what I saw, I'm going to skip forward an hour, past our training video and putting on jumpsuits...past figuring out how the helmet goes on and how to move and lift the visor.

I sat in the line waiting for my turn in the tunnel. I'd watched a few people before me, and my instructor stood in the doorway to the tunnel and beckoned me to him. I couldn't hear John Williams music. I couldn't hear anything, frankly, beyond the roar of the wind tunnel. I stood in the "falling" position, and simply leaned forward into the tunnel. My instructor caught me and helped me adjust my body position as the "driver" of the tunnel adjusted the windspeed to figure out precisely how much air we needed beneath me.

And then, he let go. And for a glorious moment I hovered there. Above the ground. In midair. I was Supe—*Oh, wait, he's adjusting my waist position. He wants me to bend my knees slightly. Relax? How do I relax? I'm flyyyyying!*

Because of the deafening sound in the wind tunnel, we had earplugs in, so all communication was done through a series of four hand signals that we were vigorously trained and tested on in the ten minute "training seminar". Before I knew it my first minute was up and I was being guided to the door of the tunnel. I grasped it and tried to stand, finding my feet simply hit the ground beneath me. I landed! I flew and then landed!

It was exhilarating but also disappointing. I hadn't felt like I soared. More like I floated. As I sat watching everyone else take their minutes, I tried to figure out how to capture the feeling I wanted to get.

All at once it was my turn again. This time, my instructor pointed up and I nodded vigorously. I wanted to do the "high fly". After a few seconds of adjusting and floating, my instructor grabbed my shoulder and my waist and lifted his feet off the ground. Together we spiraled upwards at an alarmingly fast rate. Faster than I expected. After a moment's shock, I realized we were soaring above the tunnel. And circling. And now, finally now, I was flying. I actually felt tears streaming down my face.

Since that day I've already been back a few times and know I'll go again, because each time they teach me a new trick or two (like how moving your hand slightly makes you turn, or accidentally bending your leg at the wrong moment makes you shoot up in the air so fast your coach has to grab you before you hit the ceiling). And they were right. The longest single flight I've done so far is one minute forty seconds, which frankly was more than enough to feel. It's a hard workout on your body because you're responsible for muscle contractions and keeping your position steady. It's harder than it looks.

But for that 1:40 I flew my ass off. And the second time, once I relaxed, even above the roar of the wind, I heard John Williams.

CHAPTER 32

Selfie King

"Who do you think you are, a Kardashian?"

This is a common refrain in my world these days. You see, as I mentioned before when we talked about clothing, I take every opportunity I possibly can to take a selfie. Or a picture with friends. Or have friends take a picture of me. Or court staff. Or strangers. Anywhere, anyone, anytime. It's an unusual feeling for me...oh wait hang on.

Snap!

Okay. Selfie done. Now we can discuss them.

For years I took vacation and holiday family photos, but usually I was behind the camera taking them. Rarely did I appear in them by choice. When I had to take professional photos I did my best to enjoy them but never really liked the way I looked. I didn't even like taking them when I was in happy situations, like my wedding photos.

I decided after the surgery that I needed to document the entire process for myself (also for the *Survivor* video I would be making later) and so I took photos and videos as often as possible post surgery.

About two months after surgery while out for a walk, I snapped a selfie, and a strange thing happened. I liked how it looked. I smiled in it. I felt the sun on my face. It was an amazing feeling in general. I was able to use an app on my phone to put the photo side by side with one of me taken the day of surgery. I could see the difference. Dramatic and true.

I found that selfies were not only useful for documenting the changes in me, but they boosted my self esteem. It was a successful moment. And success breeds success. Each one that looked better or different than the last drove me to take the next. Every new shirt or pair of pants needed to be documented. It became something I did without even thinking about it on such a regular basis my friends just came to accept it without thinking.

"Oh, Jonathan's just taking another selfie. Give him a second."

Usually that refrain was followed by a sigh and an eyeroll of some sort and then a good natured smile. I know I was being annoying. And frankly, still am. Yet I still do it. As often as I please.

It's important when you're going through a change or progression towards a goal to find a way to document it. Studies (that I'm sure I've read but am now citing without evidence or citation) have shown that people who document progress towards life goals—especially documentation in tangible form such as photos or written notes—are much more likely to succeed.

How much more likely? Hey, my business is anecdotes not statistics (said the guy who researched how likely he was to die on the table and quoted statistics to you earlier in the book).

Speaking of which, embracing change and evolution has also become a hallmark of my journey. Not just physically, but emotionally and mentally. For instance, I used to quote statistics to you and now I just tell you things I know will succeed and hint at things that make it seem to have scientific validity.

Sufficed to say, selfies are okay. Chronicling your journey is not only okay but in fact necessary in many instances to get the kind of success you really want. Not because it will affect your success, but because it will affect your mindset, which will truly affect your success.

CHAPTER 33

Holidays and Sweets

Christmas and Hanukkah are my favorite times of year. Actually from about Thanksgiving until Valentine's Day is my favorite patch. A time when holiday decor abounds and we're all a little kinder and happier (Scrooge notwithstanding). And of course there's the food. You thought I was going to mention family and love didn't you? Yeah, there's that too. But the food was always such a huge part of the production of the holidays to me that they're essentially inseparable. With savory dishes and cookies and desserts and frostings and more, food was just always a part of life. Especially growing up with Italian and Jewish heritage. These people know how to enjoy themselves some holidays, my friends.

As I approached the end of the summer and October loomed large in my mind, now some six months post surgery and having made significant changes and progress towards my goals, a question popped into my head.

"How the hell am I going to do the holidays?"

It was a true conundrum for me. I wanted to celebrate my successes as well as my family and bring people together at a time when, frankly, many of us needed something to cheer us up (having just survived the 2016 US Presidential Election. Oh yeah, thanks for nothing cryotubes). I wanted to host and be the glue that held my friends and family together and created joy for everyone.

I wanted to share the feeling I've had inside me and the happiness and joy I could feel welling up there. And I wanted to cook like nobody's business. But then I would want to eat, too. And eating at the holidays, although not solely responsible for my weight, sure as hell didn't help. Because I couldn't say when. I just ate until I was stuffed and in some instances overstuffed. This was my first holiday season since meeting my sleeve and I was a little worried that my sleeve might end up being a grinch.

But being a host and sharing in the things you love doesn't mean overindulging. Hadn't I learned that when baking with my daughter already? Hadn't I survived a bite of brownie and some zucchini bread? But this was different. This was a whole holiday spread. And I was going to go all out. I was going to recreate my Italian grandmother's Christmas Eve feast of the seven fishes (which for her included about 2 or 3 fishes, but God didn't mind apparently). Additionally, the first night of Hanukkah (which I also celebrate) happened to fall on Christmas Eve that year, so double bonus.

Here was the menu I'd planned for Christmas Eve Dinner:

Caesar Salad (with homemade dressing and anchovies because I'm not a heathen)
Garlic Bread

JONATHAN DICHTER • 142

Toasted Walnut Pasta in oil with cheese
Baked Giant Stuffed Clams on the half shell
Celery and Olive Salad
Potato Latkes with sour cream and apple sauce

Oh yeah...and a few desserts:

Fresh baked Ruglach (a wrapped cookie with sugared dates inside)
Dom Deluise's Sister Ann's Cookies
Russian Tea Cakes
Butter cookies (fresh baked-not from a tin)
Struffoli (deep fried Italian dough balls the size of peas smothered in honey sauce and sprinkles)
Godiva chocolates

I'll wait while you google Ruglach, the Sister Ann Cookies, and Struffoli to see what they look like. Ambitious as well as tasty. There was no way I could actually eat it all, right? But I was determined to eat it with my eyes and nose as much as I possibly could. Besides, I could have a bite of this and that couldn't I?

It's hard when you're faced with your old life and your new life. You've known how you've been for so long and you've combatted that life so hard with so much strength that you really feel good. But when those moments of "old" thought pop up, it's hard to resist them.

Thankfully my sleeve was in fact a grinch. But not the grinch who hated Christmas, and not the grinch who loved it. It was the grinch who gave little Cindy Loo Who (who was no more than two) a glass of water and patted her on the head. The one who loved that child just a smidgen enough to see that she was a sweetheart, but still had his goals in mind.

In other words, my sleeve actually let me indulge a little at a time. And I managed to do so without any major issues over the holidays. No weight gain to speak of and really nothing I couldn't eat. I just ate a little of it all. A bit of this. A taste of that. Until my sleeve said "you're done."

It helped me immensely. It helped me realize that leaving comforts behind isn't permanent. And that you can learn very easily how to live and work within your own goals while still pushing forward. And nibbling on cookies from time to time.

CHAPTER 34

Dumping at Improv Class

I was mopping sweat off my head (it was pouring off me) and I was quite literally seeing double. My head was spinning even as I sat down. I thought I was going to die. None of the people around me even noticed anything wrong for several minutes.

I'm a student of improv comedy. I started taking classes around 2016, and as of writing this I am in an advanced class where we perform for a live audience once a week. I've been cast in shows and collaborated with experienced improvisors. I've co-created and directed a show of my own. It's one of the things that is most thrilling and invigorating to my soul at this point.

Before class it's not uncommon for me and some friends to stop and get a bite to eat or a drink or coffee or, in most cases, a smoothie. Now I won't out the purveyor of the smoothie in question except to say that their name rhymes with Mamba Moose. In any event, one evening about eight months post surgery, we stopped for our smoothies before class. I was used to getting one that was primarily fruit and some veggies. No yogurt or sugar syrup base.

This night I decided I wanted to try something different. Something with a yogurt base. Same caloric content as what I was used to, so I was sure it wouldn't affect my weight loss goals. It was quite yummy. I didn't realize there was a problem until about two hours later.

We'd gotten to our break mid-class. I had noticed that the classroom seemed quite warm to me. Warm wasn't something I was used to feeling lately. In fact, more often than not I found myself chilly. This was quite an unusual feeling for me, as I'd spent nearly three decades being way too hot (that happens when you're wearing a 160 pound overcoat).

But now I was hot. Overheated in fact. I went into the restroom to use it, and realized my shirt was soaking through with sweat. I grabbed a towel to mop my brow. As I tried to focus and figure out what the problem was, I realized I was having trouble stringing a coherent thoughts together. Words in my mind literally weren't working for me at that moment. I just knew I needed to sit—and fast—or I was liable to fall down.

I grabbed some extra towels and went back into class. I sat down at the back of the room and not a minute too soon, for as soon as I sat, the room was spinning. I put my head down and closed my eyes. When I tried to open them and look around me, I was seeing blurry and double. I had no idea what was happening, but something in my mind told me it would pass if I just let it. I breathed through it and waited.

An important note about dumping syndrome: You may recall that early in my process I had a nausea-based bout of dumping syndrome after eating some mashed potatoes. This was, in fact, dumping. But a massively different kind of dumping. Let's talk about why dumping syndrome happens. If you push concentrated or refined sugars through your stomach too fast, they "dump" into your intestines without being fully digested or absorbed. Your body simply gets a massive concentrated sugar spike, and your blood sugar goes haywire.

If you don't know what effects that can have on a person, ask a diabetic about diabetic shock. Some of the symptoms of a late dumping attack can be: disorientation, body sweats, body tremors, nausea, vomiting, double vision, and a general feeling like your body is going to curl up and die.

Early dumping has to do with starches that are more pure. This is what happened with the potatoes. Late dumping, on the other hand, are sugars usually mixed with other things. Like fruits. Or vegetables. In a Mamba Moose smoothie for instance. As an aside, after this incident I did some internet research on a variety of boards for weight loss surgery patients and learned that Mamba Moose is quite the common cause of late dumping attacks. Sure enough, they were the ones that did me in.

After about ten minutes (which seemed more like three or four lifetimes) of suffering, I felt a hand on my shoulder. My friend, Lindsey, whispered to me, "You okay?"

I shook my head, no.

"What do you need?"

"Just sit near me."

And she did. I don't recall much about that class except to say that as 30-45 minutes went by, I started to regain the opportunity to focus slightly. After class we walked (albeit slowly) to a nearby restaurant where I was able to get some protein (chicken strips) in me. I couldn't take much in, but as I ate I felt my body returning to normal slowly but surely.

The sweating stopped. My vision cleared. My thoughts became coherent. I learned a valuable lesson as well. It's critical to learn what works well in your new life and what doesn't. Even if it seems harmless, it may not be. But sometimes you'll only find out by getting knocked on your ass by a Mamba Moose smoothie.

CHAPTER 35

Walt Disney World

Alright, I'm a big giant Disney nerd. I always have been. I grew up going to Walt Disney World about once every year and fell in love with the story telling, the artistry, and the theme parks and movies. Flash forward to my adult life and you'll find that my home is decorated with Disney fine art, I own a time-share at Walt Disney World, and I co-host a popular Disney podcast (hey All About the Mouseketeers! Thanks for reading!). I honeymooned at Walt Disney World, and have been back several times a year since.

But those trips were getting increasingly hard. In fact, as you know, I'd already chosen to simply hermit myself in my hotel room on one of them and never leave the room, never see the parks, and never ride a ride.

In February 2017, I was finally excited about a trip again. I was going with my daughter for a week during break. This trip was significant for me in several ways.

1) It was the first trip I'd taken to Walt Disney World since my surgery and I was down over 150 pounds already. I was quite anxious to see what it was like and what was new.

2) It was the first trip I'd take to Walt Disney World that was just me and my daughter. No mama. No grandma. No babysitter. Just my seven-year-old and me.

This trip presented some fun challenges and exciting possibilities. I was super excited to see how it was going to feel. But I'll admit I was also afraid and hesitant, because what if? What if nothing was different? What if my feet hurt? My back? My legs? What if I still couldn't fit into certain rides and attractions? What if I let my daughter down and she wasn't proud of me?

In essence, the new me was terrified that the old me was still the one going on the trip.

This is a common occurrence I've found. We find ourselves still slaving away to the fears of our past lives. We know things have changed and we know we're not the same as we once were, but we don't internalize that enough to truly believe in ourselves and the change. We're convinced that one mistake will send us spiraling backwards or worse yet—we'll find out we weren't as far along as we thought.

So what do we do in those instances? What can we do? What should we do? Well I had literally no option but to just suck it up and give it a try. My daughter deserved her Disney trip and by golly we were going to have it together. One of the things I chose to do in order to prepare myself was pack several boxes of protein snacks and bars to bring with me. I wanted to have the fuel I needed because I wasn't sure how eating theme park food was going to hit me. Or if I'd need more than I was able to get from the food inside the parks.

I went shopping and bought some new shorts and short sleeve shirts for the trip. This was one of the first moments I started to believe something might be different. I was used to wearing 3XL or in some cases 58-60 inch waist pants and shorts. Instead, I bought 38 inch waist shorts...and they fit. They were snug, but not tight. They just...fit. Like the vests and hats I'd started to like to wear with my suits to court. And to perform improv. And I was starting to believe I looked good. I was certainly starting to feel good. Maybe something was different here. Looking your best and feeling your best are truly things that once you can get them in sync can and will change everything for you.

As soon as we boarded the plane and got seated, I took the opportunity to take a selfie with her (because, selfies), and realized in that moment that we'd be taking a lot of pictures together on this trip.

The week was a blur of fun and excitement, but there were some highlighted moments I want to point out to you. These are the moments I'd been working towards. These were the stuff life and dreams and wonderful memories are made of— the successes and the emotional high points. I challenge you to find them in your daily struggles. Find those moments and burn them into your memory. Write them down. Tell stories about them. Blog. Take selfies. Celebrate every single success you have. Write a book if you like. I did.

I have a travel bag I bring with me when I go to Walt Disney World. It includes things like Desitin, mole skin and blister bandaids. You see, on average, on a good day at Walt Disney

World you might walk eight or ten miles or more through the day. The blister bandages are to help when you have blisters. The moleskin is to help avoid them when you have hot spots on your feet. The Desitin (diaper rash cream) is for...well... chafing. I have used each of these products on every Disney trip since 2006.

Until this one. Not one blister. Not one rash. No side stitches or shin splints. No hot spots. No back pain, even when carrying my kiddo on my shoulders. It was as if I was doing things for the very first time. In fact every step of the trip felt like new. No matter where we went or what we did, for the first time in my life, I wasn't the tired one. I was wearing my daughter out.

There's a newer ride in the Magic Kingdom: The Seven Dwarves Mine Train. It's a rollercoaster. It's designed for families, so it's not so scary as some other roller coasters. It swings a little from side to side as it moves which is pretty cool. I've ridden it before. It involves individual lap bars that come down around your knees and hold you in. You ride side by side and have your own lap bar.

This is not a ride that is designed for comfort. It's short enough as rides go to be okay being a tight squeeze. In fact, I've had to literally squeeze extra hard to get into the seats and work my way onto the ride.

But not this time. This time I sat comfortably and even had room to spare. Nothing about the ride was uncomfortable. I smiled so broad I thought my face would split in half. I remember a single thought when I got off the train. "This is what thin people feel like, isn't it? I'm one of the skinny people now."

I didn't see people looking at me as the "fat guy" or the "big guy". When people complimented me on my shirts (I wear some fun ones), I didn't feel it was a compliment to the fat guy with the cool shirt. They were just seeing a guy.

I saw a shirt I liked in a store called MouseGear. It's the largest gift shop in EPCOT. It was cool, and I hadn't bought any clothing yet on this trip. In previous trips I'd been a shopping machine—artwork, souvenirs, housewares, and yes, clothing. Anything I could find that was XXXL I'd buy because it was Disney and it would be tight, but fit. I had avoided it this time. I wasn't sure I wanted to try on Disney clothes. They're notoriously tight fitting.

But I liked this shirt. I wanted to try it on. I grabbed the first one on the rack and took it back to the dressing room, honestly without looking at the size. I was pretty sure it was an XL. I slid it on with my daughter standing there beside me so she could tell me how it looked. It seemed to fit. She agreed. It was a little form fitting in the shoulders, but it draped well and really, frankly, looked good on me. I was happy with the fit. So I took it off to buy it.

And saw the label. And the letter "L" staring at me.

Large. I was wearing a Large. Not an Extra-Large. Not an XXL or an XXXL. I'd not only dropped numbers from in front of XL, I'd dropped the letter X entirely. I felt my breath catch slightly and sat down in the dressing room.

"Daddo? Are you okay?"

"Yeah, kiddo." I heard a shake to my voice.

"Why are you crying?"

"I'm happy, Kiddo. I'm so so happy."

My final bill that day at MouseGear was over $650 in brand new L clothes. I bought damn near everything I could get my hands on. As I grabbed clothes I told every cast member I could find that I was buying clothes smaller than I'd ever worn in my adult life before. My kiddo joined in the fun and started grabbing clothes off shelves and finding me things that would fit.

"Oh wait. Not that one, Kiddo."

"Why not, Daddo?"

"Sweetie, Daddo isn't so much into princess shirts."

"But it's a large."

Well, she was right about that one. But we did leave it behind.

Despite eating a little nibble of everything my daughter ate and ordering whatever pleased me, I actually came home from that trip having lost a full pound. Because even though I was enjoying life, I wasn't over indulging, and I was managing to integrate my new body into my new life. And it was working.

CHAPTER 36

Survivor Video (Tribe)

In January 2017, I was cast in an improv comedy show called "The Tribe Has Spoken," which was an improvised version of a popular reality show on a desert island. Each week we would compete in improv and physical challenges and then vote each other off the show in front of a live audience at voting council. While a "performance", it was entirely real. There were chances for immunity, challenges, alliances, betrayals, blindsides, and more. It was one of the most thrilling, fun experiences I've ever had performing, to date.

Far more than that, however, it was the perfect bookend to my *Survivor* audition video. You see, I'd been recording ten to fifteen seconds every few weeks/months since before the surgery. And as I edited the video together into a final cut, I was able to watch the progress I made.

I watched me pre surgery. I watched me announce my registration for the RunDisney event. I watched me getting on a bicycle for the first time in 20 years. I watched my weight drop below 300 pounds. Then below 250. I watched as I exercised and got fitter. And I watched as I became new.

Becoming seems to be the theme of my video. Becoming and transformation. I had become a better version of myself. Not the best version, but a better one. Why not the best version? Because the best version of ourselves is always the next version. The one we're striving for. We can be an amazing version of ourselves, but the moment we stop striving to be more, we become complacent. We slip back into our old ways of thinking and believing and before we know it, our habits are starting to reform. We run the risk of unbecoming. Untransforming.

I'm not saying that I'm ultra diligent and never make mistakes. Hell, I just ate a boatload of tiramisu and gelato while on vacation in Italy (more about this later). But I nibbled. I enjoyed and indulged. I did so while I was walking through Italy and learning the history of another country and without pain or fear or soreness in my body. I was striving to be and do more. I was using my transformation to try to move forward.

That's what it's about. That's what being a *Survivor* is and why the show was so important to me. It's not about a chance to win a million dollars, although that sort of money demands attention. No. To me *Survivor* is the ultimate challenge and the ultimate test of whether or not I've truly become more than I've ever been. It's my litmus test.

In February 2017 I submitted my video. To date, I've heard nothing in return. However, a friend of a friend put me in touch with someone who works as a consultant for the show. She has nothing whatsoever to do with casting, but I did ask her if she was willing to watch my audition video.

"Let me know when they call you."

"They haven't yet."

"They should. If they don't, keep resubmitting this video every three to four months until you hear from them. They work with certain themes and casting ideas and it may just be that you're not the right guy for this season. Or your video hasn't gotten in the hands of the right production assistant."

"Okay. But you think it's good?"

"Like I said. Let me know when they call you."

They still haven't. But I'm updating my video. And will resubmit it. Soon. And often. Until they call me. And they will. Because I'm a *Survivor* already. I just need the show to catch up to me.

CHAPTER 37

Tempers - Business Increases - Letting Go

I'm a lawyer. I handle criminal defense work, primarily DUI and driving related crimes. This is a high stress job, but as you may have guessed from my writing, I have a decent attitude about life and humor, so it rarely gets to me. Or rather, it didn't.

You see, about eight months post surgery I had new pictures taken of me, and updated my website with a lot of new information. We did a complete website overhaul. As a result of that, a newfound confidence, and some intangibles, my business started to pick up. It continued to pick up over time. Within a few months, I was busier than I'd ever been.

I'm all about attention to detail and have a small touch of OCD. In other words, I'm a micromanager. There is very little that goes on at my office that I don't give my personal attention to or lay hands on. At the time, I had an office manager, but when it came to handling my clients and their legal woes, that was all me. If it wasn't me, I got a little jittery and worrisome. I know I'm a quality attorney and have the skills my clients need and want. It's why I've been as successful as I've been.

But by the time January had arrived, my caseload had nearly doubled in size. I was working longer hours and pushing myself at every opportunity. I was burning the candle at both ends and although my eating was good, my exercise was essentially nonexistent. I didn't have time.

My patience was growing thin. I found myself getting crabby in general. With friends. With my office manager. With colleagues.

Finally...with Elizabeth. I was grouchy and snapping at her. She started to notice and, God bless that adorable little girl, she called me out on it. She actually had the nerve and courage to ask her dad why he was a little shorter of temper than normal. Now, let me be clear, I wasn't shouting at her or being violent. But I was short tempered and I didn't like it. Not one little bit.

I assured her that it was just work stress and that as time went by it would ease and that I would be able to rest a little bit and get back to normal. Maybe a vacation—our Disney trip— would help. It did. Temporarily. But the stressors and difficulties I had were still waiting for me when I got home.

I had two choices. Go on as I had been.

Or let go of some control. I decided to hire an associate attorney. I decided to trust someone with my clients and my practice. After an exhaustive search of people who were willing and able to work for me, I selected an associate. I was afraid of not being able to afford it or them running my practice into the ground. Terrified in fact.

As I said, I'm a micromanager. Giving someone control over those parts of my world was something I hadn't ever considered doing before. It was something I've said in the past I'd never ever do. But now I'd done it.

Let's talk about control. Control is something we all strive for, and if you're a Type A personality like I am, control is one of the ways you find yourself safe and able to manage your world. It's also something that's holding you back. Trust me, I know.

One of the things you need to be able to do as you move forward in your life journey and through whatever changes you're going through is just to let go of a little bit of that control. Not all of it, but enough that you have the time and energy you need to still be you and focus on the things that make you unique. If your focus is being pulled every direction but the ones that are most important to you, you can't possibly be of any use to anyone. Especially yourself. Ultimately it will be your downfall.

My best friend, at reading these words, I'm sure is shaking her head and wondering who actually wrote them because they're so antithetical to who I am and my very personage. I've come to learn, however, just how true it is. Some say "let go and let God." I choose to leave the divine out of it and simply say "let go and let's go". What I mean is that in order to move forward, you may have to just give up a little bit of what's been holding you back.

For me that meant trusting someone to handle my clients. Hand picking them. Training them. Observing them. And then letting them fly on their own. You see, one of my idols, Walter Elias Disney, had the same working model.

Hire the best people you can to do the job you need done. Then get the hell out of their way and let them do it. Did he still retain control and management? Of course. But he didn't micromanage every single moment.

Within days of hiring my associate I was already feeling less stressed. More relaxed. More "me". And that feeling is what truly allowed me to push myself to the next level and will aid me to do the same as I move forward.

CHAPTER 38

The Dark Side Challenge

In July 2016, only two months post surgery, I committed my-self to getting back into doing long distance races. The specter of my last race was looming in my mind throughout my decision. The last race I'd done was a RunDisney half marathon in 2011 (not counting the one in 2016 that I'd registered for but chose not to even attempt during my retreat).

Flash forward to July 2016. I decided I was going to slay this demon once and for all. But not for about a year. I registered for the RunDisney Walt Disney World Dark Side Challenge in April 2017. This is not just one race, but two. A 10k on Saturday and a half marathon on Sunday. A grand total of 19.3 miles of redemption. I knew what I needed to do and I *would* do whatever I had to in order to complete this challenge.

Sadly, I had more heart for training than time. And although I exercised regularly and was active, my formal "training" was very lax. As April approached I started to worry quite a bit. Especially since I'd committed to a second event in 2017— this time in November at Disneyland in Anaheim, California. I'd heard that this year marked the 10th anniversary of what they call the "coast-to-coast" challenge where, if you do a half marathon in Walt Disney World and in Disneyland in the same calendar year, you get a special medal. So I figured I might as well do it right and registered for the RunDisney Infinity Gauntlet challenge in November. Another 10k/half marathon combination challenge. Needless to say I was starting to get worried because I hadn't been "formally" training.

As you know, in February I took my daughter with me on a vacation to Walt Disney World. My first trip there since surgery. I tracked my activity through the trip and was happy to see that I was walking seven to ten miles per day and had no blisters, no shin or knee pain, no back pain, and no complaints. It was the first time I can remember being comfortable on a trip like that. I've already mentioned some other fun firsts on that trip in a previous chapter, but needless to say, it heartened me a little. And all at once it was April and I was alone on a plane headed to Orlando again. Despite being alone on the trip, I was happy that my dear friend Jerry and his mother were also joining me in the races. Both would be there with me on the course.

My first full day there was spent at the race expo, which is a place where, along with 35,000 of your closest friends, you fight your way through a crowd to get a flimsy piece of paper and pin it on your shirt while you walk an ungodly distance. It's also a place where you can buy new gadgets that you never thought you needed and will invariably try out on the race and decide midway through that you never should have bothered with in the first place and *who the hell invented these things anyway and why is the new water bottle leaking iced tea all over your hands which are now stained brown?*

The bus to the expo was supposed to leave our hotel at 9:30am. I was there at 9:15. With a large group of other athletes (side question: Did I just refer to myself as an athlete? Wow. There's a first, and I think I mostly meant it) we sat and waited. 9:30 no bus. 9:45 no bus and a bigger crowd. Finally at 9:50 I mentioned to the couple I'd been chatting with that I was headed to the lobby to get a cab. They happily joined me. When we arrived at the lobby, there was a mom and her son who also wanted a cab. We decided to share. A van pulled up for the five of us when six more people walked over and asked if they could all share with us. Runners and Disney people are pretty much uniformly approachable and friendly, I've found, so of course we all piled into the van. The driver looked at me, riding shotgun with wide eyes.

"Woah. How many people are in this van?" I looked back and counted. We were up to twelve. Clearly we'd exceeded the maximum allowable number of people in the van.

"Three," I said.

He nodded and took off with us to the expo.

Once there, I got my packet and my race shirts (the super awesome tech shirts we all get for doing races). This is a good moment to stop and talk about some frustration and anxiety I had regarding these shirts and their sizes. I was wearing larges. But not in the tech shirts. Oh no. I got larges. But found out later that the larges were a little too snug. So I exchanged them for XLs. Which felt so much like a failure. So I tried on some standard Disney large shirts. They fit. Except one. It was too big. So I bought a medium. I complained in an online forum about the inconsistency in sizing for shirts at this point, and how now had to try on shirts that I intended to wear. The overwhelming response I got was: "Try being a woman." Apparently this is an ongoing frustration, but one I had just discovered. The frustration of never quite knowing what your actual size was, which gets even more challenging for a while after weight loss surgery. In any event, I digress.

After a day taking it easy at the parks, and engaging in some dancing with cast members, I found myself awake at 3am before the 10k, hanging out in the race corrals. These races started at 5:30am so that we'd be done by the time the parks actually opened. As I sat in the corral getting ready for the race, I found myself very nervous. What if I failed? What if I got swept? What if...hold on. I steadied myself. I'd pushed myself to get here and I was some fifty pounds lighter than my fastest race before. Sure. But the Large shirts hadn't fit. I was double talking and doubting myself harder than I had in a long while. Before I knew it, we were shuffling from our race corrals towards the start line. My headphones were on and it was time.

I started a nice fast walking pace and just kept going. The 10k is something of a blur. It took about 90 minutes and it was a bit uneventful overall. It served as a great warm up for the half marathon, however. I was so proud of my medal. But truth be told I was terrified about the half marathon. My legs were tired. Not sore, but tired. My mind wasn't sure if I was ready for it. But I had no choice. It was time to do this and redeem myself. I found the success of the 10k both motivational and inspirational.

The first five miles of the half marathon were relatively normal. I tried to stay with Jerry and his mother, but they managed to out pace me about two miles in. Still, I kept them in sight as long as I could. Regardless, I was doing my race at my pace. Periodically I would look behind me to see if there were people and to check for the balloon ladies. Never saw them.

Eight miles in, after going through Disney's Animal Kingdom, I saw a site that nearly stopped me in my tracks. An overpass. From World Drive. To EPCOT. The very spot where I was swept in my last half marathon. I was approaching it. It was around 7:30am. The clouds were starting to burn off and I felt the first rays of the Florida sun on my face. My headset clicked to a new song and I heard the familiar piano notes that start Idina Menzel's version of "Let It Go." As I began climbing the overpass and hearing the music with the sun on my skin, I sang that song along with the music at the top of my lungs.

"I'm never going back. The past is in the past!" Tears were streaming down my face. I had conquered this moment. It felt amazing. But there were still five miles to go.

Ten miles into the race I was approaching Disney's Hollywood Studios, and I hit the wall. Anyone who's done a long distance race will tell you that, around three quarters of the way through, you can hit a wall physically and mentally where your body just literally seizes up and doesn't want to keep moving. I hit it hard. My doubts and fears took over. I was done for. I couldn't possibly do this. I'd never succeed. I was still the fat guy who couldn't get down the hallway without getting out of breath. My muscles burned and ached. My mind was starting to bog down with negativity.

Then a string of images and words flooded my mind. Facebook comments from my group telling me how proud people were of my initial success, how much they liked excerpts from this book. Hugs and words of pride from my best friend. The video of well wishes and "good lucks" that she put together for me to watch just before beginning the race (seriously Jen, that was awesome. One of the best things ever.) Trying on a vest for the first time and it fitting well. New pictures for my website. My daughter, Elizabeth, wrapping her arms around me telling me she could get them all the way around now. Elizabeth in the pool telling me how good she thought I looked. Elizabeth and I riding bikes for the first time together. Elizabeth and I walking. Playing. Running. Smiling. Laughing. Riding Seven Dwarves Mine Train. Elizabeth.

My daughter's strength and willpower, love, devotion, and belief flowed into me like gas to an empty tank. Like Popeye eating that can of spinach. Pac-Man biting into a power pellet. The grinch's heart growing three sizes. I could go on with examples and awful metaphors, but you get the idea. I was energized and revitalized. I balled my fists and listened to the music when "King of Pride Rock" from the Lion King hit. I was climbing Pride Rock ready to roar and become that King, like I was always supposed to be. And my daughter had helped push me that extra step when I needed it.

The finish line grew in front of me at mile thirteen and I actually stepped up the pace and ran. I was giddy and leaped across the finish line, finishing the half marathon in 3:30:02. I got my medals and emotion poured out of me. When I calmed down and saw Jerry and his mother and made my way out of the finish area, I called Elizabeth immediately, to tell her how much she'd helped me. That we'd actually succeeded together.

Truly that's my hope for you. That we succeed together. I doubt I'll be that energy source for you in that moment when you hit your wall, physical, mental, or what have you, however, my sincerest hope is that our journey together through this book allows you to tap into whatever sources you have for that energy spike. To grab hold of what you need and keep moving forward to finish your goals.

Then set new ones.

My next race was in November 2017 when I went to Anaheim for another RunDisney event and beat that 3:30:02 time by over fifteen minutes. After that, who knew what I was capable of? And isn't that truly the most amazing feeling?

Epilogue: Italy

As I write this, I am sitting in seat 2E on my first ever flight with British Airways. In fact, this is my first ever flight to Europe. It just turns out that my mother and I have decided to take a mother son trip for Mother's Day and we'll be touring Italy.

The fact that I have boarded this plane one year and three days from my surgery is not lost on me. It's the symbolism of what I've accomplished and struggled with (and continue to do so). Regardless, I'll say that this trip feels like the culmination of a long journey that began a long time ago—one that will propel me to my future and marks the occasion properly.

We'll check into the Hotel Grand Melia in Rome later today and begin an adventure through Italy that will be unlike any trip I've ever taken before. Not because it's Italy, although there's that, but rather because I get to be healthy and changed and new here, and anywhere really that nourishes my soul, which I know this will. And I can't wait.

Grazie, boungiornio! And Ciao!

Acknowledgements

There are so many people to thank for helping not only this book, but this transformation to take place.

Obviously, my mother, Kay, is a huge part and I cannot thank her enough for the gift. As she loves to remind people, she "gave her son life, twice." I love you, Mom!

My daughter, Elizabeth. I just love you so much.

My editor, best friend, fellow-author and surgery support person, Jennifer DeLucy, who stood by me through ups and downs in life as well as authorship, but never once gave up on me. Jen, you're literally the best.

My medical team: Dr. Catherine Zeh, Dr. Robert Landerholm, Dayna Pitsch and everyone at Eviva! You guys are artists and helped me so much. I can't thank you enough.

In addition to Jennifer, many other friends who are authors lent their ears and eyes to this project. GG Silverman, Jeanie Gallo, Kimberley Bouchard. Thank you so much.

The subtitle for this book was the result of a contest I held inside a Facebook group. The winning suggestion was an amalgam of three peoples suggestions. Rupa, Amy, and Erin-

you guys did a great job and the subtitle absolutely captures this journey!

Lastly, my sincerest thanks to my advance and beta readers. Andi, Jennifer, Jeanie, Shari, Robin, Mike, Marcy, Sara, Tain, Karen, and April. You guys rocked it!

ABOUT THE AUTHOR

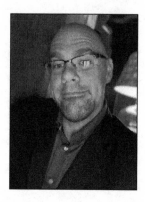

Jonathan Dichter is an author, lawyer, father, speaker, actor, magician, podcaster, half-marathoner, and unashamed geek. His sincerest hope is that this book has somehow inspired you to transform into your best self. Please reach out and tell him your story!

www.sleevelifebook.com

11012159R00115

Made in the USA
San Bernardino, CA
02 December 2018